Introduction to Epidemiologic Research Methods
IN PUBLIC HEALTH PRACTICE

Susan L. Bailey, PhD
Assistant Professor of Public Health
Benedictine University

Deepa Handu, PhD, RD, LDN
Director, Dietetic Internship, Edward Hines Jr. VA Hospital
Adjunct Professor of Nutrition, Benedictine University

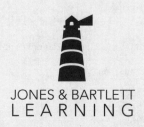

JONES & BARTLETT
LEARNING

World Headquarters
Jones & Bartlett Learning
5 Wall Street
Burlington, MA 01803
978-443-5000
info@jblearning.com
www.jblearning.com

Jones & Bartlett Learning books and products are available through most bookstores and online book-sellers. To contact Jones & Bartlett Learning directly, call 800-832-0034, fax 978-443-8000, or visit our website, www.jblearning.com.

Substantial discounts on bulk quantities of Jones & Bartlett Learning publications are available to corporations, professional associations, and other qualified organizations. For details and specific discount information, contact the special sales department at Jones & Bartlett Learning via the above contact information or send an email to specialsales@jblearning.com.

Introduction to Epidemiologic Research Methods in Public Health Practice is an independent publication and has not been authorized, sponsored, or otherwise approved by the owners of the trademarks or service marks referenced in this product.

This publication is designed to provide accurate and authoritative information in regard to the Subject Matter covered. It is sold with the understanding that the publisher is not engaged in rendering legal, accounting, or other professional service. If legal advice or other expert assistance is required, the service of a competent professional person should be sought.

Some images in this book feature models. These models do not necessarily endorse, represent, or partici-pate in the activities represented in the images.

Production Credits

Publisher: Michael Brown
Editorial Assistant: Kayla Dos Santos
Editorial Assistant: Chloe Falivene
Production Assistant: Leia Poritz
Senior Marketing Manager: Sophie Fleck Teague
Marketing Intern: Shayna Goodman
Manufacturing and Inventory Control
  Supervisor: Amy Bacus

Composition: DiacriTech
Cover Design: Michael O'Donnell
Cover Image: © fotoecho/ShutterStock, Inc.
Printing and Binding: Edwards Brothers Malloy
Cover Printing: Edwards Brothers Malloy

Library of Congress Cataloging-in-Publication Data
Bailey, Susan.
  Introduction to epidemiologic research methods in public health practice / Susan Bailey and Deepa Handu.
        p. ; cm.
  Includes bibliographical references and index.
  ISBN 978-1-4496-2784-3 (pbk.) – ISBN 1-4496-2784-6 (pbk.)
  I. Handu, Deepa. II. Title.
  [DNLM: 1. Epidemiologic Research Design. 2. Public Health Practice. WA 950]
  614.4072—dc23
                                2012009651

6048

Printed in the United States of America
16 15 14 13 12   10 9 8 7 6 5 4 3 2 1

Table of Contents

Acknowledgments

We both wish to thank the nine anonymous reviewers of our manuscript. Their comments and suggestions made a significant contribution to the quality of the final product.

I (Dr. Bailey) also wish to thank my research mentors over the course of my education and career. These include Dr. Nicholas Danigelis, who first lured me into the research world as an undergraduate at the University of Vermont; Dr. Peter Marsden, who whipped me into shape as a graduate student at the University of North Carolina at Chapel Hill; Dr. Robert Bray, who modeled extreme patience with the research process at the Research Triangle Institute; and Dr. Lawrence Ouellet, who got me into the field in Chicago's Westside.

I (Dr. Handu) want to extend my greatest gratitude to all my mentors and my students, without whom I would not have realized my love for teaching. On a personal note, a big thank you to my husband and my two kids (6 and 2 year olds) for their love and patience during this project.

Preface

You are reading this preface for one of two reasons: (1) your instructor has chosen this text for your class on research methods, or (2) you are considering choosing this text as a resource or guide for your own research study. This text is written to serve both purposes. Details about research procedures are presented in a way to educate you as a student and to serve as a road map for you as a researcher to navigate the options, limitations, necessary assumptions, and realistic expectations of your research study. Take a deep breath and move through the process systematically.

If you are a novice researcher, your most important goals are to determine what is possible in your study (overreaching is a common problem for the inexperienced investigator) and to focus on doing everything possible to conduct the strongest study in terms of validity. More simply, the best initial lesson is to learn how to make the absolute best of what is available to you.

Most likely you have some background in research as a student, or perhaps as a research assistant on a study being run by someone else. In this case, you need the bigger picture of an entire study, from formulating the research question to reporting the results. This book is meant to serve as a guide for you to conduct your own study, whether a research project for a class, a thesis or dissertation or capstone, or an independent investigation as part of your career.

The study questions and exercises at the end of chapters are intended to be used for these two different purposes: At one level, the exercises are pedagogic with the goal of learning and applying new information. On a more advanced level, the exercises are intended to stimulate the development of your own study details from beginning to end.

The overall focus of this text is on quantitative methods in the field of epidemiology. Quantitative studies are not the only type of studies useful in epidemiology, but they are the primary designs for a field of study developed to "count things"—outbreaks, deaths, injuries, and diseases. As such, it is expected that you have some general knowledge about statistics or biostatistics and about epidemiology as a field. We do review the basics of these areas, but for the purpose of choosing and initiating the use of them, not learning them anew. Throughout the book, you are given suggestions of books to consult for more detail about concepts and procedures that may be somewhat new to you.

A potentially useful analogy is to think of this book as a cookbook. The necessary ingredients are listed and the procedures explained to prepare a dish or a component of a research study. The novice researcher, like the aspiring chef, will follow the recipes exactly to the letter to maximize the probability of preparing a successful dish or conducting a successful study. With experience, both the veteran researcher and professional chef know how to adapt recipes (studies) to the tastes of diners (research audience), the available ingredients (money, time, research subjects, measures), and the appropriate possible procedures (sampling techniques, retention procedures, analysis plans). Occasionally, the experienced chef consults the cookbook when she wishes to refresh a technique or prepare a new dish. Likewise, this book can be used as a reference for researchers who wish to use a new study design or statistical technique.

Unlike culinary projects, research studies rarely come out exactly as anticipated. The researcher rarely has as much control over the details of her study in the real world as does a chef over the cooking process. Especially when studying people, it is impossible to anticipate every aspect of the study. You may get a smaller than anticipated sample. Your follow-up sample may be biased in unexpected ways. There may be a confounder you did not think to measure. With knowledge of the research process and experience with it, you will learn to anticipate and prevent likely problems and address and hopefully overcome the unlikely ones.

About the Authors

Susan L. Bailey, PhD is an Assistant Professor of Public Health at Benedictine University in Lisle, Illinois, where she teaches biostatistics, epidemiology, and research methods in the master of public health program. Her more than 20-year professional career has been devoted to public health research. Dr. Bailey has numerous publications in professional journals, including the *American Journal of Public Health, American Journal of Epidemiology, Journal of Health and Social Behavior, Journal of Studies on Alcohol,* and *Journal of Acquired Immunity Deficiency Syndrome.* She has served on the editorial board of the *Journal of Health and Social Behavior* and as an ad hoc reviewer for many journals. Dr. Bailey has also served as Principal and Co-Investigator on several NIH and CDC R01 grants and as a reviewer on numerous NIH grant review committees. Her general areas of research interest are risky health behaviors among adolescents and the risk of HIV and HCV infection among young injection drug users. She began her career at the Research Triangle Institute in North Carolina, where she received hands-on training in the conduct of research, from question to publication of results. Dr. Bailey's research focus at this time was adolescent drug and alcohol use. She then served as a Research Assistant Professor of Psychiatry at the University of Pittsburgh Medical Center, where she studied substance use disorders among adolescents. Before accepting her current position at Benedictine University, Dr. Bailey served as a Research Associate Professor of Epidemiology and Biostatistics at the University of Illinois at Chicago. In this role, she was the Research Director of the Community Outreach Intervention Projects, a service and research effort serving and studying injection drug users in Chicago.

Deepa Handu, PhD, RD, LDN holds a doctoral degree in human nutrition (Michigan State University, 2005) and a master's degree in food science and human nutrition (Maharaja Sayajirao University, India, 1997). Before joining

Edward Hines Jr. Hospital, Department of Veteran Affairs as the Director of Dietetic Internship in 2011, Dr. Handu taught nutrition and research courses at Benedictine University and Loyola University in Chicago.

Dr. Handu's research interests lie in the areas of public health nutrition, youth overweight prevalence and obesity risk, and diabetes. Dr. Handu has been involved in school-based intervention programs to reduce the prevalence of obesity and encourage the idea of healthy lifestyle. She has also been involved with Chicago public schools vending machine task force and has been a founding member and cochair of research for the FORWARD initiative to lower childhood obesity in DuPage County, Illinois.

Dr. Handu has delivered presentations at national professional conferences, and as coauthor of many research studies, she has a number of publications to her credit and several works in progress. Dr. Handu was selected as a 2009 Recognized Young Dietitian of the Year by the Illinois Dietetic Association. She is a past recipient of the following grant awards for research activities: Consortium to Lower Obesity in Chicago Children (2006); African American Family Initiative Project Grant (2003); Blue Cross Blue Shield Student Research Award (2001); and Council on Renal Nutrition Grant, National Kidney Foundation (2000).

CHAPTER 1

Overview of the Research Process

LEARNING OBJECTIVES

By the end of this chapter the reader will be able to:
- Explain the steps in the research process.
- Describe the basic components of each step.
- Use the steps as an organizing mechanism for a research project.

CHAPTER OUTLINE

I. Introduction
II. Definition of Research
III. Research Process
IV. Conclusion

Scientific research consists of seeing what everyone else has seen, but thinking what no one else has thought.

—Unknown

INTRODUCTION

The main purpose of this chapter is to provide an overview of the research process. Many students quiver at the thought of conducting research, but, in reality, each of us conducts research projects in our everyday lives. For example, buying a car involves the research process. The process involves collecting data to decide between a new or used car, makes and models, and amenities; to consider budget limitations, dealer locations, their inventory, and prices; and so on. Data are collected and analyzed to answer the question: "What type of car best meets my needs and budget, and where is the best place to buy it?" This is the research process.

DEFINITION OF RESEARCH

Research is a systematic process based on the scientific method that facilitates the identification of relationships and determination of differences in order to answer a question. The scientific method is a process that uses an organized structure to formulate questions and determine answers in a research project. The key steps of scientific method are:

1. *Generate a hypothesis or ask a research question.* Research ideas usually start with a vague understanding of some problem. This understanding is usually based on one's readings, observations, or other experiences in day-to-day life. In this step, the researcher usually refines the research question or hypothesis so that it is focused and testable.
2. *Observation or data collection.* The types of data and methods to collect them are determined by the research question. Methods of data collection include surveys, questionnaires, anthropometrics, observations, and so on.
3. *Testing the hypothesis through data analysis.* This step involves analyzing the data to draw conclusions to support/refute the hypothesis or answer the research question.
4. *Conclusions.* Results of the analysis are interpreted vis-à-vis the hypothesis or research question.
5. *Compare the results to previous established theory.* The findings from the research are compared to the established theory to determine whether or not they "fit" or support the theory.

RESEARCH PROCESS

Regardless of the area of research or choice of methodology, the research process involves similar activities. The process is an expression of the basic scientific method using the following steps: statement of the problem, generating a hypothesis, review of relevant studies, creating measures, choosing the sample, collecting data, analyzing data, and reporting results. **Figure 1–1** illustrates the research process.

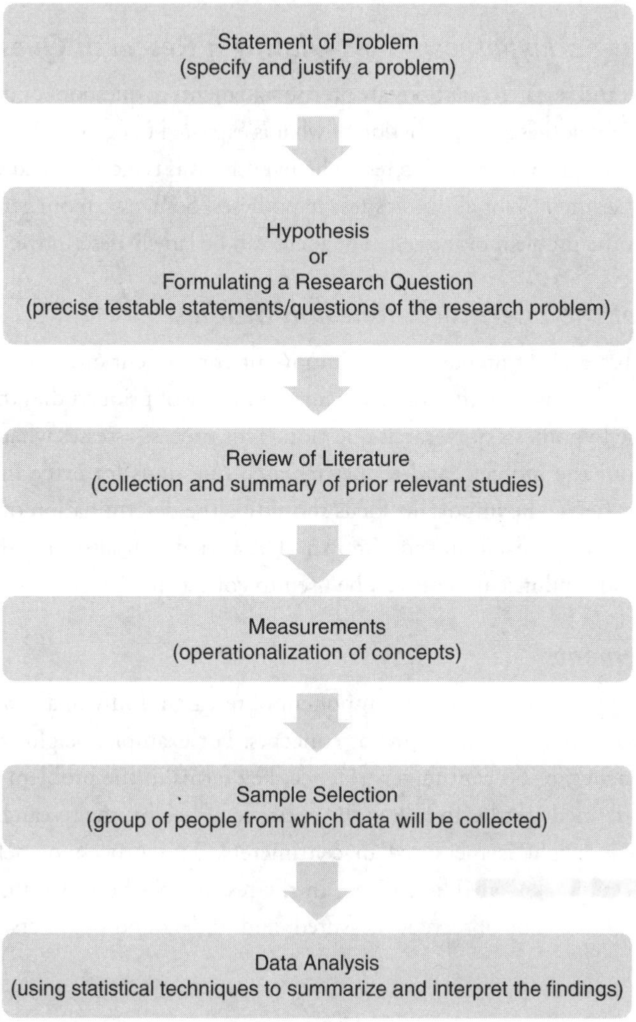

Statement of Problem
(specify and justify a problem)

Hypothesis
or
Formulating a Research Question
(precise testable statements/questions of the research problem)

Review of Literature
(collection and summary of prior relevant studies)

Measurements
(operationalization of concepts)

Sample Selection
(group of people from which data will be collected)

Data Analysis
(using statistical techniques to summarize and interpret the findings)

FIGURE 1–1 Illustration of the Research Process

Statement of the Problem

The first step in research is pinpointing the topic of interest. Researchers usually start out with a vague idea of some problem and then slowly try to refine this idea into a concise statement. They review studies relevant to this topic to further illuminate the problem and refine the research question. A strong problem statement is one supported by a thorough review of relevant study results and a strong rationale or justification for performing the study. How will this study advance the field of interest?

Generating a Hypothesis/Formulating a Research Question

Hypotheses and research questions are precise statements or questions of the research problems. A hypothesis is a prediction of what is expected to occur, or a relationship expected between concepts of interest. The hypothesis is typically tested with some form of experiment. Not all studies test hypotheses. Some ask more general questions about the problem of interest. The focus can be largely descriptive.

Review of the Literature: Relevant Studies

A thorough search of literature is an important component of the research process. The review involves the collection and summary of prior studies that are relevant to the hypothesis or research question. This process assesses what is already known about the problem and refines research questions for extending knowledge in this field. The important focus should be the determination of what this study will add to what is already known. The review can also provide ideas of what methods and instruments can be used to collect the data.

Measurements

Measurements are an important component of research. Individuals vary in their interpretations of particular terms or concepts. For example, height = 60 could mean 60 inches, or 60 centimeters. Hence, key terms in the problem statement should be defined clearly. To follow the example of height, the researcher should indicate that height is measured in centimeters. This process of definition is called operationalization: The concept in the researcher's head is translated into something that can be observed, measured, and understood by others.

Sample

If the study involves human subjects, then *sample* means a group of people from which data will be collected (subjects of the study). If the study is analyzing secondary data collected by another investigator, then *sample* refers to the data sets.

Usually the sample is a group of people representing a target population, and the population is the larger group to whom the results are to be generalized. Types of research bias or systematic errors can be avoided with precise definitions of the target population and rigorous sampling strategies.

Instrumentation

Instruments are tools that collect and measure data. The selection of the tool depends on the focus and type of research study (case study, observational study, cohort, and so on) being conducted. Each tool that will be used to collect data should be as precise (reliable) as possible and measure the intended concept (validity).

Data Analysis

This step in the process involves the use of statistical techniques to summarize and interpret relevant research results. Basic descriptive statistics (i.e., measure of incidence and prevalence, central tendency, dispersion) are part of every quantitative research study. Inferential statistics are used in studies that test hypotheses. The main objective of data analysis is to answer the research questions or test the hypothesis. Based on analysis results, conclusions are drawn and interpreted in the context of previous studies.

CONCLUSION

This chapter illustrates research as a process of generating questions, selecting samples, and measuring, collecting, and analyzing data to answer questions. Commonly used terms in research (e.g., statement of the problem, hypothesis, review of literature, and so on) are introduced in this chapter. The information presented in this text is comprehensive, but not particularly detailed. Readers are encouraged to consult other sources for more details about specific procedures in the research process.

FURTHER READING

Chatburn, R. L. (2011). *Handbook for health care research* (2nd ed.). Sudbury, MA: Jones & Bartlett Learning.

Clark, V. L. P., & Creswell, J. W. (2010). *Understanding research: A consumer's guide.* Upper Saddle River, NJ: Pearson Education.

Drew, C. J., Hardman, M. L., & Hosp, J. L. (2008). *Designing and conducting research in education.* Thousand Oaks, CA: Sage Publications.

McMillan, J. H. (2008). *Educational research: fundamentals for the consumer* (5th ed.). Boston: Pearson Education.

CHAPTER 2

Research Goals in Epidemiology

LEARNING OBJECTIVES

By the end of this chapter the reader will be able to:

- Use the research goal as the organizing principle of a study design.
- Distinguish between general research goals.
- Explain the requirements for causality.
- Realize the practical limitations of a research goal.

CHAPTER OUTLINE

What is the meaning of life?

INTRODUCTION

Well, that question is probably better suited for a philosopher than an epidemiologist. To determine appropriate research goals in epidemiology, significance, scientific rigor, and feasibility are key considerations. Questioning the meaning of life is certainly significant in terms of importance to humankind, but designing a study to answer this question is decidedly not feasible in terms of scope, time, and cost; and a rigorous scientific design, given the scope of this question, would be impossible.

Starting with a question that is not feasible or even possible to answer illustrates how the research goal is the organizing principle for every element of the study. In this chapter, we will review the feasible epidemiologic research goals as well as their practical limitations.

TYPES AND EXAMPLES OF RESEARCH GOALS

We will start with the least ambitious and most limited type of goal and move to the most ambitious and least limited research goal. Within the context of the overall substantive goals of epidemiology as a field, a limited and less ambitious goal is not a compromise of practical significance. Description is usually the first step in the quest for causality.

Descriptive Research Goal

A descriptive research goal is intended to "describe" a health phenomenon in terms of its distribution across person, place, and time. The goal is not to test a hypothesis about the causes or even correlates of the phenomenon. Rather, the value of a descriptive study is to gain information necessary to formulate a hypothesis. This goal is appropriate for emerging or rare diseases or health problems about which little is known. It is also useful for monitoring and tracking diseases over time.

Incidence and Prevalence

The health phenomenon under study can be anything that compromises human physical and mental health, from cancer to infectious diseases, and from drug abuse to traffic injuries. The health problem is typically measured as incidence and prevalence. Briefly, incidence is the number of new cases of disease or death during a specific period of time out of the total population at risk for the disease or death. The population at risk can be either the number of subjects without the disease at the onset of the study (cumulative incidence) or the total number without the disease multiplied by their time at risk during the study period (incidence density or incidence rate). Prevalence is the number of existing cases of disease or deaths out of the total population of interest. Calculating incidence or prevalence is a basic, but very important component of a descriptive study.[*]

Person, Place, and Time

Beyond incidence and prevalence, a descriptive study could focus on the "who, when, and where" (person, time, and place) of the health phenomenon of interest. Characteristics of the person with the health problem include sociodemographic characteristics, such as age and gender, as well as other characteristics, such as general health status, or risk factors (like cigarette smoking) that may be relevant to the disorder. Characteristics of time include the hour, day, week, and so on of an outbreak, as well as collective measures of time like historical periods, cycles, and trends. Characteristics of the place where the health problem occurs include geographic, geologic, climactic, and similar criteria. In the case of outbreaks, specific buildings or similar localized areas would be the focus. The goal of descriptive research is to gather "clues" about the concentration of health phenomena among specific populations, during particular times, and localized in key areas. Ideally, these clues suggest potential causes and, subsequently, hypotheses to be tested and interventions to be evaluated.

Example: Obesity Research

Technically, childhood obesity in the United States is an epidemic (the prevalence and incidence is higher than what would be expected historically) with its beginning increase in the late 1970s (Ogden, Carroll, Curtin, et al., 2010). The increase in prevalence since 1971 is shown in **Figure 2–1**. These results are an example of a descriptive study with a focus on the timing of the disease or condition. The unexpected increase in prevalence among children and adolescents, and even among adults in the United States was alarming enough to stimulate additional descriptive and analytic research on obesity.

Focus on the person characteristics of childhood obesity shows that Hispanic boys and non-Hispanic black girls are at increased risk for obesity (Ogden et al., 2010). More focused person-centered research on adolescent obesity shows that

---

[*]For more detailed information about incidence and prevalence, see *Essential Epidemiology: Principles and Applications* by William Oleckno (2002) and *Epidemiology for Public Health Practice* by Robert Friis and Thomas Sellers (2009).

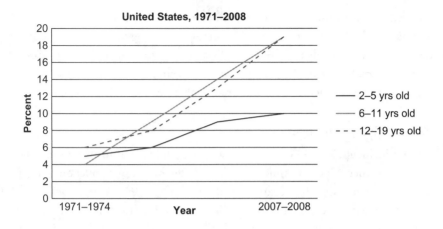

FIGURE 2–1 Increase in Childhood Obesity

Source: Data from Ogden, C. L., Carroll, M. D., Curtin, L. R., Lamb, M. M., & Flegal, K. M. (2010). Prevalence of high body mass index in US children and adolescents, 2007–2008. *Journal of the American Medical Association, 303*(3), 242–249; AMA Publishing Group © 2010.

adolescents with autism and Down syndrome have an exceptionally high prevalence of obesity (Murray & Ryan-Krause, 2010; Rimmer, Yamaki, Lowry, et al., 2010). These descriptive results stimulate a focus on potential cultural, genetic, and biological causes of obesity in these subgroups of adolescents, as well as identify these groups as appropriate target populations for prevention and intervention.

We move to Canada for an example of a descriptive study of obesity that focuses on clustering and comparisons of prevalence by place—urban and rural. The Canadian Heart Health Surveys Research Group (Reeder, Chen, Macdonald, et al., 1997) compared obesity prevalence in nine Canadian provinces from 1986 to 1992. They found no urban–rural differences in obesity for men and women in all provinces except those in western Canada. In western Canada, rural men and women are more likely to be obese compared to their urban counterparts. These results stimulate research to pinpoint the reasons why there are rural–urban differences in western Canada and indicate a need for tailored intervention programs in this region of Canada.

Association Research Goal

A next important research goal in epidemiology is to determine factors that are associated with or related to morbidity and mortality. This type of study typically moves beyond person, place, and time comparisons to comparisons based on potential risk factors for disease and death.

Risk Factors

Risk factors are exposures that are associated with a disease (Friis & Sellers, 2009). Exposures can be a vast array of experiences such as contact with an infectious agent, behaviors including high-fat diet and excessive alcohol use, contact with environmental poisons, and conditions of life such as crowded housing, low income, and stress. Risk factors are especially relevant for epidemiologic research because the etiology of most diseases is a complex combination of causes and potential causes. For many practical and empirical reasons, the relationships between risk factors and disease onset cannot always be shown to be causal. For example, as reviewed later in this chapter, coronary heart disease has been associated with a number of risk factors, including elevated serum cholesterol, high blood pressure, obesity, and cigarette smoking (Kagan, Kannel, Dawber, et al., 1963).

According to Friis and Sellers (2009), an exposure that is associated with a disease or other health problem can be considered a risk factor if it meets the following criteria:

1. There is a dose-response relationship—the higher the level or intensity of the exposure, the higher the probability or severity of the disease.
2. Temporality of the exposure and disease are appropriate—the exposure precedes the onset of the disease in time.
3. The observed relationship between exposure and the disease is not due to some source of error in the design or conduct of the study.

These criteria are a subset of the criteria needed to establish causality, as discussed later in this chapter.

But like most things in life, the identification of risk factors is more complicated than simply demonstrating a relationship between exposure and disease onset. Robust results are those that consider potential sources of error in relationships, as well as other factors that may influence the significance, strength, or direction of relationships between an exposure and disease.

Measures of Association or Effect

In epidemiologic studies, measures of association test relationships between exposures and outcomes. These measures are used in studies focusing on associations and those testing causal relationships (effects). Their interpretation depends on whether certain criteria for causality are met (discussed shortly). The measures are best understood in the context of contingency or two-by-two tables with the exposure reported in the rows and the outcome in the columns. **Table 2–1** shows an example contingency table, as well as formulas for the most commonly used measures.

Table 2–1 Two-by-Two Table Showing the Relationship Between an Exposure and an Outcome

		Outcome		
		Has outcome	Does not have outcome	*Total*
	Exposed	a	b	a + b
Exposure	Not exposed	c	d	c + d
	Total	a + c	a + d	a + b + c + d

Risk Ratio $= \dfrac{[a/(a+b)]}{[c/(c+d)]} = $ [prevalence or incidence of outcome for the exposed group] divided by [prevalence or incidence of the outcome for the unexposed group]

Risk Difference $= [a/(a+b)] - [c/(c+d)] = $ [prevalence or incidence of outcome for the exposed group] minus [prevalence or incidence of the outcome for the unexposed group]

Odds Ratio $= \dfrac{(a/c)}{(b/d)} = $ (exposed divided by unexposed for those with the outcome, or cases) divided by (exposed divided by unexposed for those without the outcome, or controls)

Attributable Risk $= \dfrac{[a/(a+b)] - [c/(c+d)]}{[a/(a+b)]} = $ Proportion of the prevalence or incidence of the outcome for the exposed group that can be attributed to the exposure

Population Attributable Risk $= \dfrac{[(a+c)/(a+b+c+d)] - [c/(c+d)]}{[(a+c)/(a+b+c+d)]} = $ Proportion of the total prevalence or incidence that can be attributed to the exposure

The purpose of all of these calculations is to measure how strongly the outcome is associated with or attributable to the exposure. They can be calculated by comparing incidences or comparing prevalences of the outcome. Risk ratios and risk differences (called rate ratios and rate differences for comparisons of incidence densities) are used in cross-section and cohort study designs, and odds ratios are used in case-control studies. Attributable risk (AR) and population attributable risk (PAR) are descriptive measures showing the proportion of the incidence or prevalence of the outcome that is attributed to (or the result of, or explained by, or associated with) the exposure.[*]

Confounding

Confounding is present when a third factor or variable distorts the relationship between an exposure and disease (Rothman, 1986). The distortion can take the form of erroneously inflating or deflating the strength of the association between the exposure and disease. Consequently, confounding is often a form of systematic error

---

[*]For more detailed information about measure of association, see *Essential Epidemiology: Principles and Applications* by William Oleckno (2002) and *Epidemiology for Public Health Practice* by Robert Friis and Thomas Sellers (2009).

or bias. Reporting an association between exposure and disease without testing for obvious or even potential confounding in the association is a biased study and result.

Testing for confounding involves comparing the magnitude and even direction of the simple association between exposure and outcome (crude association) with the adjusted association when the potential confounder is included in the analysis. Confounding is present when the following criteria are met:

1. The confounding variable has an effect, either as a risk factor or cause, on the disease.
2. The confounding variable has an effect on the exposure, independent of the disease.
3. The confounding variable does not intervene in time and the causal chain between the exposure and disease. In other words, the exposure does not influence the confounding variable.

Figure 2–2a illustrates these criteria of associations.

Although not epidemiologic, the following example provides a clear illustration of confounding. A city planning intern noticed that there is a dose-response relationship between the number of fire trucks present at a fire and the amount of property damage at the site of the fire. Specifically, the greater the number of fire trucks, the greater the amount of property damage, as illustrated in **Figure 2–2b**.

The intern proposes to his preceptor that efforts should be made to limit the number of fire trucks called to a fire in order to limit the amount of property damage. The preceptor suggests that the intern study this relationship by observing several fires and measuring any feasible relevant factors associated with property damage. **Figure 2–2c** illustrates the results of the study.

Confounder

Exposure   Disease

FIGURE 2–2a Illustration of the Criteria for Confounding

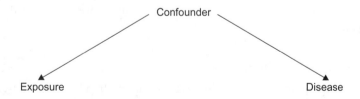

Number of Fire Trucks ⎯⎯⎯⎯⎯⎯⎯⎯⎯⎯→ Property Damage

FIGURE 2–2b Relationship Between the Number of Fire Trucks and the Severity of Property Damage

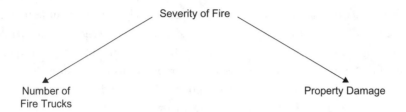

FIGURE 2–2c Severity of the Fire Confounds the Relationship Between the Number of Fire Trucks and Amount of Property Damage

The intern was able to show that the association between the number of fire trucks and property damage was very weak and not statistically significant when the severity of the fire is considered by examining the associations between trucks and damage for mild fires, for moderate fires, and for severe fires. In addition, he found that the severity of the fire influences both the number of trucks called to the fire and the amount of property damage due to the fire. Subsequently, the intern withdrew his original proposal.

Confounding can be controlled or prevented in all stages of the research study. In the design or planning stage, potential confounders can be included in the measures planned for data collection. In the sampling stage, subjects can be randomly selected or randomly assigned to groups in order to minimize systematic differences between groups and between those selected and not selected for the study. Other preventative sampling measures include matching characteristics between study groups and restriction (limiting or excluding) based on the confounder. Finally, in the analysis stage, analyses can be conducted within stratification or grouping based on the confounder, or multivariate models including the confounder can be tested.

Effect Modification (Interaction)

While an unrecognized confounding relationship can be a bias in a study, effect modification, also called interaction, is a meaningful result. Effect modification is present if the strength or direction of the relationship between exposure and disease differs for subgroups of a third factor, such as gender or age group (Hennekens, Buring, & Mayrent, 1987). The demonstration of effect modification adds additional information about the association between exposure and disease onset.

For example, an investigator determines, in a hypothetical study, that a measure of association between lead exposure and brain damage has a value of 5.0 (a quite strong relationship). Because she also hypothesizes that the risk of lead exposure for older children with brain damage would be greater than that for infants with brain damage, she examines the relationship between lead exposure and brain damage separately for infants (younger than 1 year of age), preschool children (ages 1 to 4 years), and young school children (ages 5 to 9 years). She finds that the measure of association is 2.0 for infants, 4.5 for preschool children, and 6.0 for young school children. She concludes that the risk of lead exposure increases by age among children with brain damage. In other words, age modifies the effect of lead exposure on brain damage. Again, this is a hypothetical result.

The presence of effect modification can be tested in two general ways. As was done in the hypothetical study, the data can be stratified or grouped according to categories of the potential modifier and the association between exposure and disease determined within the groups, then compared across the groups. Second, an interaction term, essentially multiplying the exposure by the modifier, can be tested in multivariate models.

Example: The Framingham Heart Study

> This, then, is what has been called the coronary profile, a picture of the individual most prone to develop coronary heart disease. With some of these features still subject to confirmation, he may be described as a mesomorphic, obese, middle-aged male, with high serum cholesterol, high blood pressure, low vital capacity, and an abnormal electrocardiogram. He eats too much of too rich foods, smokes cigarettes to excess, and is physically inactive both in occupation and in recreation. He is ambitious, aggressive, and subject to frequent deadlines and other emotional stresses. The closer an individual comes to fitting this pattern, the greater should be the efforts of his physician to alter, where practicable, these characteristics of the patient and his environment (Kagan et al., 1963, p. 893).

Much of what we know currently about the risk factors for cardiovascular disease (CVD) has been demonstrated in a long and ongoing history of studies collectively known as the Framingham Heart Study. The study began in 1948 in response to the shift in the 20th century from infectious diseases to chronic disorders as the leading causes of death in the United States. At this time, CVD emerged as the leading cause of death.

More than 5,000 adults aged 30 to 62 years and free of CVD were recruited for the study in Framingham, Massachusetts. Framingham was chosen as the study site because its residents numbered high enough to provide the desired quota of subjects, were relatively heterogeneous in ethnicity and socioeconomic status, and were stable in terms of limited out-migration (Feinleib, 1983). Subjects returned to the study every 2 years for medical examinations and testing. In 1971, their adult children were enrolled in the study. In 2002, their adult grandchildren were recruited to participate. In addition, another group was enrolled in 1994 to reflect the growing ethnic and socioeconomic diversity of Framingham (Framingham Heart Study, 2012). As the study has progressed, the research goals have also expanded to include examinations of health phenomena beyond CVD.

In addition to the risk factors for CVD summarized in the quotation on the previous page (Kagan et al., 1963), Framingham studies have found associations in the form of risk factors between menopause and CVD (Gordon, Kannel, Hjortland, et al., 1978), use of oral contraceptives and both hypertension and thromboembolism (Kannel, 1979), chronic atrial fibrillation and stroke (Wolf, Dawber, Thomas, et al., 1978), cigarette smoking and reduced levels of high-density lipoproteins (HDL) (Garrison, Kannel, Feinleib, et al., 1978), diabetes and CVD (Kannel & McGee, 1979), combined use of oral contraceptives and smoking and thrombosis among women 35 years and older (Castelli, 1999), and chronic cough and myocardial infarction (Haider, Larson, O'Donnell, et al., 1999). Identified protective factors against CVD include higher levels of HDL (Gordon, Castelli, Hjortland, et al., 1977) and moderate alcohol use (Kannel & Ellison, 1996).

Confounding and effect modification have also been demonstrated in the Framingham studies. A perplexing negative relationship between low body weight and elevated mortality in men was found to be confounded by cigarette smoking (Garrison, Feinleib, Castelli, et al., 1983). Cigarette smoking leads to both low body weight and elevated mortality among men. However, more recent studies of the relationship between low body weight and mortality have demonstrated a relationship independent of cigarette smoking (Woods, Iuliano-Burns, & Walker, 2011). Many cases of effect modification have also been shown, usually modification by gender and age. The relationship between higher serum cholesterol and CVD among men is modified by age in that the increase in risk is sevenfold among men younger than 50 years of age, but only two-and-one-half-fold for men age 50 years and older (Kagan et al., 1963). There is an association between gout and CVD for men, but not for women (Abbott, Brand, Kannel, et al., 1988). Among men, Raynaud's phenomenon (a circulatory disorder) is associated with age and with smoking, but among women, it is associated with marital status and alcohol use (Fraenkel et al., 1999). These results may be due to differences in the prevalence of behavioral factors between genders rather than true causal mechanisms. Among men and women younger than 65 years, Type A behavior and emotional lability are associated with CVD for women, but worries about aging are associated with CVD for men (Haynes, Feinleib, Levine, et al., 1978). As the Framingham tradition continues, these and many more proven associations have led to hypotheses, both tested and untested, about the causes of CVD and other health phenomena.

Causal Research Goal

The ultimate goal of epidemiologic research is to determine the causes of morbidity and mortality. Confidence that a factor is truly a cause depends on a rigorous study design, repetition of studies showing the same result, and adherence to strict criteria developed through centuries of research by scientific thinkers, including Robert Koch and Jakob Henle (Evans, 1976), Sir Austin Bradford Hill (1965), and Mervyn Susser (1977).

Validity and Reliability

Although a valid and reliable study is the ideal for all research goals (descriptive, association, causal, evaluation), accuracy and precision are vital to make inferences about causality. Confounding bias in a relationship between exposure and disease would compromise the status of an exposure as a true cause. A sample that does not adequately represent the target population to which results are generalized (lack of external validity) compromises the inference that the exposure is a cause in the presumed context. A potential cause that is not accurately measured cannot represent a true cause no matter the strength of the relationship between exposure and disease. Bias and error in study design and conduct compromise the ability to conclude that an exposure is an actual cause of morbidity or mortality.

The Scientific Method

A discussion of the scientific method is particularly informative in the context of appreciating what is required to infer a causal relationship. The method has its roots in ancient Egypt and Greece with substantial refinements and expansions made by Muslim scientist al-Haytham in the 11th century, Francis Bacon and René Descartes in the 17th century, and John Stuart Mill in the 19th century.

Figure 2–3 illustrates a modern conceptualization of the necessary steps in the scientific method.

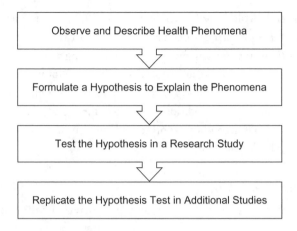

FIGURE 2–3 Steps in the Scientific Method

Note that the first step in the scientific method, to observe and describe health phenomena, is the goal of descriptive epidemiology described earlier in this chapter. The requirements for a causal research goal include the remaining steps of formulating, testing, and retesting hypotheses. Suppose we observe that sickle cell anemia is more common among African Americans compared to other racial or ethnic groups. Naturally, we begin to hypothesize about the reasons for this observation. Our hypothesis might focus on genetic factors unique to African Americans. Perhaps we would focus on environmental factors or cultural factors or some combination of these. Next, we would test our hypothesis by designing a study to obtain a sample that is representative of African Americans and to measure with optimal validity and precision candidate genes, prevalence of potentially relevant factors (such as exposure to malaria) in the historical environment, and whatever else we hypothesize to be relevant. Not only do we strive to design a valid and precise study, but also one that is replicable by other investigators and in other contexts. Every aspect of our study must be empirical or observable and measurable. The greater the number of subsequent studies that replicate our results, especially in different contexts such as multiple study designs, alternative but still precise measurements, and various samples of African Americans, the stronger our case for a causal relationship.

Criteria for Causality

In 1882, Robert Koch demonstrated the "germ theory" of disease by specifying disease organisms as the causes of specific diseases. With later refinement of the theory by Jakob Henle in 1887, the Henle-Koch postulates were developed in an effort to prove the pathogenesis of disease (Evans, 1976). They specified that the infectious agent must be:

1. Present in every case of the disease;
2. Isolated and grown in pure culture;
3. The cause of the disease when introduced into a healthy host;
4. Recoverable and grown again in pure culture; and
5. The cause of no other disease.

These criteria are relevant for explaining infectious diseases, but infectious diseases are only part of the focus of epidemiology. They do little to guide the discovery of the causes of chronic diseases, which are the predominant causes of death in contemporary developed countries.

An expanded set of criteria for determining causality was outlined in medical statistician Sir Austin Bradford Hill's President's Address to the Section of Occupational Medicine of the Royal Society of Medicine in 1965 (Hill, 1965). This seminal address identified nine criteria that are applicable to causality in epidemiologic research:

1. Strength of the association between exposure and disease. A strong association is less likely to be due to bias or random error.
2. Consistency in observing the association in multiple investigations. Ideally, the additional studies should be conducted by multiple investigators examining the potential association in various contexts of places, circumstances, and times.
3. The association is specific to particular persons, places, times, and/or health phenomena.
4. The exposure precedes in time the development of the disease. If this particular criterion is not met, there is no point in further investigating the possibility of causality.
5. Dose-response or biological gradient in linear relationships. The greater the exposure, the greater the risk of disease.
6. Plausibility. It is biologically possible, at least within the current knowledge of biology, that the exposure can cause the disease.
7. Coherence. The association makes sense given what is known about the biology and natural history of the particular disease.
8. Experiment. Causality is more plausible when the investigator is able to manipulate the exposure and observe the results.

9. Analogy. Causality is more plausible if an association between a similar exposure and/or a similar disease has already been established.

Some of these criteria are illustrated in the following landmark epidemiologic case study.

Example: Cigarette Smoking and Lung Cancer

Together with Richard Doll, Sir Austin Bradford Hill demonstrated that cigarette smoking causes lung cancer by finding evidence that meets many of Hill's criteria for causality (Doll & Hill, 1950, 1952, 1954, 1956, 1964). This series of studies grew out of clinical observations in the 1920s that cigarette smoking might cause lung cancer. It was not until the 1964 Surgeon General's Report on Smoking (U.S. Public Health Service, 1964) that enough evidence was collected to begin convincing the general public that cigarette smoking is strongly associated with morbidity and mortality. What follows is a brief summary of research evidence in the context of criteria for causality.

1. *Strength of the association between exposure and disease.* **Figure 2–4** presents measures of association between smoking and lung cancer. These measures indicate that smokers were nearly 10 times more likely than nonsmokers to have lung cancer and 18 times more likely to die from lung cancer. More than 90% of lung cancer deaths among smokers were attributable to smoking. These associations are undeniably strong.

2. *Consistency in observing the association in multiple investigations.* In the 1950s, Doll and Hill demonstrated a strong relationship between smoking and lung cancer in two large-scale and long-term studies (case-control and prospective cohort) of British physicians. A search of the medical literature in 2011 produced 13,559 articles about cigarette smoking and lung cancer. Results of a few of the most recent studies showed that exposure to secondhand smoke increases continine (an alkaloid found in tobacco) levels among nonsmokers (Baltar et al., 2011); cigarette smoking explains more than 50% of the difference in life expectancy at 50 years between U.S. immigrants (nonsmokers) and U.S. citizens (smokers) (Blue & Fenelon, 2011); and smokers have significantly elevated white blood cell counts compared to nonsmokers (Frost-Pineda et al., 2011).

3. *Specificity.* A recent case-control study of lung cancer showed that occupational exposure to sulfuric acid (a known carcinogen) in mist form

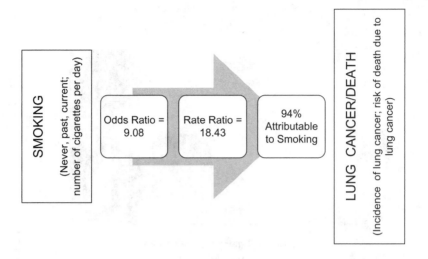

FIGURE 2–4 Strength of the Association Between Cigarette Smoking and Lung Cancer

Source: Data from Doll, R., & Hill, A. B. A study of the aetiology of carcinoma of the lung. *British Medical Journal, 2*(4797), 1271–1286, BMJ Publishing Group, © 1952; Data from Doll, R., & Hill, A. B. Mortality in relation to smoking: Ten years' observation on male British doctors. *British Medical Journal, 1*(5395), 1399–1410, BMJ Publishing Group, © 1964.

is associated with damage to the larynx, but not with lung cancer. The only demonstrated risk factor for lung cancer was cigarette smoking (Soskolne et al., 2011). These results offer some support that lung cancer is specific to cigarette exposure, but not to a similar inhaled carcinogen.

4. *The exposure precedes the development of the disease.* Doll and Hill's studies measured current or recent lung cancer and current or former cigarette use. The prospective cohort study helped to establish that a history of smoking precedes the onset of cancer. However, the temporal order is clouded by current smoking, and the long latency period between exposure and the onset of lung cancer can allow other potential causes to intervene.

5. *Dose-response.* Doll and Hill were able to provide very strong evidence for a dose-response relationship between cigarette smoking and lung cancer. **Figure 2–5** presents this evidence. These data show that the risk for lung cancer mortality increases linearly with the number of cigarettes smoked per day. Clearly, risk increases with exposure.

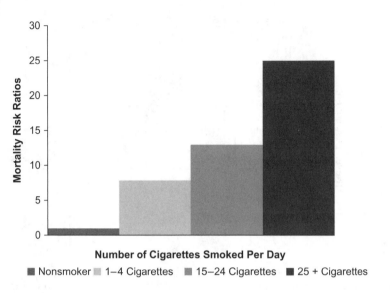

FIGURE 2–5 Relationship Between Number of Cigarettes Smoked and the Risk of Lung Cancer Deaths

Source: Data from Doll, R., & Peto R. Mortality in relation to smoking: 20 years of observation on male British doctors. *British Medical Journal, 2*(6051), 1525–1536. BMJ Publishing Group, © 1976.

Evaluation Research Goal

The most important goal of epidemiology as a field is to discover ways to prevent morbidity and mortality. Once a cause is identified, prevention efforts can be developed to eliminate or minimize the cause, thereby preventing or minimizing the health phenomena. However, even with a known and confirmed cause, the prevention program will not be effective if it does not affect the cause. The purpose of an evaluation study is to determine whether or not the program is efficacious (effective change for those receiving the treatment and not for those not receiving the treatment) in preventing the health outcome.

Ideally, the evaluation will use the traditional experimental research design with a pretest measuring the health phenomena before the intervention, a concurrent measure of the fidelity in implementing the intervention, then a posttest to measure any change in the health phenomena subsequent to the intervention. A strong design would include a control group that does not receive the intervention and random assignment of subjects into the experimental and control groups to minimize bias between groups. A strong design would also include a relatively long follow-up period to determine whether or not an effect is enduring. As seen in the following case study, studies showing that an intervention is not effective are valuable in indicating that interventions other than the one evaluated should be implemented.

Example: Evaluation of Drug Abuse Resistance Education (DARE)

> D.A.R.E. was founded in 1983 in Los Angeles and has proven so successful that it is now being implemented in 75 percent of our nation's school districts and in more than 43 countries around the world (DARE, 2012).

This school-based drug abuse prevention program was founded in 1983, and evaluation studies began in the mid-1980s. This review will focus on evaluations that used the essential features of the experimental design—control or comparison group, pretest–posttest measures, or posttest only with random assignment. These features help to minimize study bias (by randomly assigning students to the experimental or control group) and isolate effects that are due to the intervention (by comparing outcomes for those who did and did not participate in the program and measuring changes in the outcome from before to after the program).

Evaluations of the effect of DARE participation on students' drug use conducted in Illinois (Ennett, Rosenbaum, Flewelling, et al., 1994), Kentucky (Faine & Bohlander, 1989), North Carolina (Ringwalt, Ennett, & Holt, 1991), and South Carolina (Harmon, 1993) showed that DARE had negligible effects on participants' drug use. More recent studies indicated that a revised DARE had no impact on drug use among elementary school students in urban schools (Vincus, Ringwalt, Harris, et al., 2010), but a study of Tennessee schools did show that the program had an effect on preventing the initiation of cigarette use (Ahmed, Ahmed, Bennett, et al., 2002).

With such a relatively long tradition of DARE evaluation studies, it is possible to "study the studies" or "analyze the analysis" through the use of meta-analysis. Meta-analysis is a process used to summarize and even analyze the results of several evaluation studies (Sutton, Jones, Abrams, et al., 1999). Measures of intervention effects on the outcome of interest from individual studies are combined and weighted to calculate one mean effect size across all studies. In a meta-analysis of eight evaluation studies, Ennett, Tobler, Ringwalt, and colleagues (1994) calculated a mean effect size of only 0.06. Another study (West & O'Neal, 2004) analyzed 10 studies and reported an even smaller effect size of 0.01. Pan and Bai (2009) analyzed 20 studies and found a very small (within the context of relevant study factors such as sample sizes) overall effect of DARE on adolescent drug use.

DARE may be an effective program in some ways, but these evaluations show that it is likely not effective in preventing drug use among young people.

PRACTICAL LIMITATIONS OF A RESEARCH GOAL

One mistake even seasoned researchers sometimes make is to draw implications from their study results that go beyond their original research goal. A descriptive study can suggest, but not actually test the association between exposure and disease. An association study does not demonstrate causality. An evaluation study without the essential elements of an experimental design does not demonstrate the efficacy of an intervention. As a researcher and a consumer of research, particular attention should be paid to the connection of the research goal outlined in the introduction of the research article, thesis, capstone, and so on, and the implications of results drawn in the discussion section. Generalizations of results beyond the scope of the research goal have no value.

CONCLUSION

We still do not know much about the indisputable meaning of life, but we should have a better understanding of the different levels of research questions and the conclusions that can be drawn from them. Descriptive goals describe health phenomena and incidence and prevalence of morbidity and mortality in terms of the distribution of the disease among particular groups of people, in specific areas, and in focused periods of time. Association goals move to the next step of discovering additional factors that are related to the disease. Care should be taken to show that the exposure is truly associated with the outcome and the relationship is not confounded by other factors or exposures. The determination of true risk factors suggests hypotheses to be tested in causal studies to support or refute their role as the cause of disease. Ideally, causal studies identify factors that should be manipulated to prevent or intervene in the course of the disease. This is the ideal because many intervention programs are designed and implemented without knowledge of whether or not the focus of the program is even related to the outcome of interest. They are not "evidence-based." Finally, evaluation studies indicate whether or not the intervention changes the cause, thereby preventing the disease.

Studies that address these goals should be designed specifically for the goal. They should be free, to the extent possible and practical, of bias and random error.

Finally, the implications drawn from study results must be limited to the scope of the research goal. A study designed and implemented according these criteria may someday tell us the meaning of life.

VOCABULARY

Analytic goal	Exposure	Reliability
Attributable risk	Evaluation	Risk difference
Causal research goal	Evidence-based	Risk factor
Confounding	Incidence	Risk ratio
Criteria for causality	Odds ratio	Scientific method
Descriptive goal	Outcome	Temporality
Dose-response	Person, place, time	Validity
Effect modification	Population attributable risk	
Efficacy	Prevalence	

STUDY QUESTIONS AND EXERCISES

1. A businessman returns home to San Diego from a trip to China. On the way home, he had a layover in Hawaii where he visited relatives. While in Hawaii, he started to feel ill. His symptoms included respiratory problems, fever, fatigue, and vertigo. When he returned home, he suffered a seizure and died. In 1 week's time, 4 of his family members in both Hawaii and San Diego were dead, as were more than 10 people in China. As an epidemiologist at the Centers for Disease Control and Prevention (CDC), you are assigned to get to the bottom of this outbreak—quickly.
   a. What research focus should you use to begin your investigation?
   b. What factors should you examine and enumerate?

2. Continuing the scenario from problem 1, you discover that this new illness is spread easily by airborne and hard-surface contacts. From two of the victims, laboratory personnel on your team successfully isolate and replicate a virus similar to the H1N1 (bird flu) virus.
   a. What research focus should you use in your next study?
   b. What factors should you examine and enumerate?

3. Continuing the scenario from problems 1 and 2:
   a. How would you demonstrate, scientifically, that this new virus causes this new illness?
   b. How would you address the key criteria for causality?

4. Continuing this example from problems 1–3, your team has developed a promising vaccine to prevent this new illness.
   a. What research focus should you use to demonstrate the efficacy of the vaccine?
   b. What factors should you examine and enumerate?
5. If you are preparing to conduct your own research study, what research focus is most important for your research idea? Why is this focus appropriate for your study? What practical problems do you anticipate with this focus at this point in your study?

REFERENCES

Abbott, R. D., Brand, F. N., Kannel, W. B., & Castelli, W. P. (1988). Gout and coronary heart disease: The Framingham study. *Journal of Clinical Epidemiology, 41*(3), 237–242.

Ahmed, N. U., Ahmed, N. S., Bennett, C. R., & Hinds, J. E. (2002). Impact of a drug abuse resistance education (D.A.R.E) program in preventing the initiation of cigarette smoking in fifth- and sixth-grade students. *Journal of the National Medical Association, 94*(4), 249–256.

Baltar, V. T., Xun, W. W., Chuang, S. C., Relton, C., Ueland, P. M., Vollset, S. E., et al. (2011). Smoking, secondhand smoke, and cotinine levels in a subset of EPIC cohort. *Cancer Epidemiology, Biomarkers & Prevention: A Publication of the American Association for Cancer Research, Cosponsored by the American Society of Preventive Oncology, 20*(5), 869–875.

Blue, L., & Fenelon, A. (2011). Explaining low mortality among US immigrants relative to native-born Americans: The role of smoking. *International Journal of Epidemiology, 40*(3), 786–793.

Castelli, W. P. (1999). Cardiovascular disease: Pathogenesis, epidemiology, and risk among users of oral contraceptives who smoke. *American Journal of Obstetrics and Gynecology, 180*(6 Pt 2), S349–356.

Doll, R., & Hill, A. B. (1950). Smoking and carcinoma of the lung; preliminary report. *British Medical Journal, 2*(4682), 739–748.

Doll, R., & Hill, A. B. (1952). A study of the aetiology of carcinoma of the lung. *British Medical Journal, 2*(4797), 1271–1286.

Doll, R., & Hill, A. B. (1954). The mortality of doctors in relation to their smoking habits: A preliminary report. *British Medical Journal, 1*(4877), 1451–1455.

Doll, R., & Hill, A. B. (1956). Lung cancer and other causes of death in relation to smoking: A second report on the mortality of British doctors. *British Medical Journal, 2*(5001), 1071–1081.

Doll, R., & Hill, A. B. (1964). Mortality in relation to smoking: Ten years' observations of British doctors. *British Medical Journal, 1*(5395), 1399–1410.

Drug Abuse Resistance Education (DARE). (2012). *About DARE.* Retrieved February 10, 2012, from http://www.dare.com/home/about_dare.asp.

Ennett, S. T., Rosenbaum, D. P., Flewelling, R. L., Bieler, G. S., Ringwalt, C. L., & Bailey, S. L. (1994). Long-term evaluation of drug abuse resistance education. *Addictive Behaviors, 19*(2), 113–125.

Ennett, S. T., Tobler, N. S., Ringwalt, C. L., & Flewelling, R. L. (1994). How effective is drug abuse resistance education? A meta-analysis of project DARE outcome evaluations. *American Journal of Public Health, 84*(9), 1394–1401.

Evans, A. S. (1976). Causation and disease: The Henle-Koch postulates revisited. *The Yale Journal of Biology and Medicine, 49*(2), 175–195.

Faine, J. R., & Bohlander, E. (1989). *DARE in Kentucky schools 1988–1989* (unpublished report). Bowling Green, KY: Western Kentucky University, Social Research Laboratory.

Feinleib, M. (1983). The Framingham Study: Sample selection, follow-up and methods of analyses. *National Cancer Institute Monograph, 67*, 59–64.

Fraenkel, L., Zhang, Y., Chaisson, C. E., Maricq, H. R., Evans, S. R., Brand, F., et al. (1999). Different factors influencing the expression of Raynaud's phenomenon in men and women. *Arthritis and Rheumatism, 42*(2), 306–310.

Framingham Heart Study. (2012). *Omni cohorts.* Retrieved February 12, 2012, from www .framinghamheartstudy.org/participants/omni.html

Friis, R. H., & Sellers, T. A. (2009). *Epidemiology for public health practice* (4th ed.). Sudbury, MA: Jones and Bartlett Publishers.

Frost-Pineda, K., Liang, Q., Liu, J., Rimmer, L., Jin, Y., Feng, S., et al. (2011). Biomarkers of potential harm among adult smokers and nonsmokers in the total exposure study. *Nicotine & Tobacco Research: Official Journal of the Society for Research on Nicotine and Tobacco, 13*(3), 182–193.

Garrison, R. J., Feinleib, M., Castelli, W. P., & McNamara, P. M. (1983). Cigarette smoking as a confounder of the relationship between relative weight and long-term mortality. The Framingham heart study. *The Journal of the American Medical Association, 249*(16), 2199–2203.

Garrison, R. J., Kannel, W. B., Feinleib, M., Castelli, W. P., McNamara, P. M., & Padgett, S. J. (1978). Cigarette smoking and HDL cholesterol: The Framingham offspring study. *Atherosclerosis, 30*(1), 17–25.

Gordon, T., Castelli, W. P., Hjortland, M. C., Kannel, W. B., & Dawber, T. R. (1977). High density lipoprotein as a protective factor against coronary heart disease. The Framingham study. *The American Journal of Medicine, 62*(5), 707–714.

Gordon, T., Kannel, W. B., Hjortland, M. C., & McNamara, P. M. (1978). Menopause and coronary heart disease. The Framingham study. *Annals of Internal Medicine, 89*(2), 157–161.

Haider, A. W., Larson, M. G., O'Donnell, C. J., Evans, J. C., Wilson, P. W., & Levy, D. (1999). The association of chronic cough with the risk of myocardial infarction: The Framingham heart study. *The American Journal of Medicine, 106*(3), 279–284.

Harmon, M. A. (1993). Reducing the risk of drug involvement among early adolescents: An evaluation in drug abuse resistance education (DARE). *Evaluation Review, 17*, 221.

Haynes, S. G., Feinleib, M., Levine, S., Scotch, N., & Kannel, W. B. (1978). The relationship of psychosocial factors to coronary heart disease in the Framingham study. II. Prevalence of coronary heart disease. *American Journal of Epidemiology, 107*(5), 384–402.

Hennekens, C. H., Buring, J. E., & Mayrent, S. L. (1987). *Epidemiology in medicine* (1st ed.). Boston: Little, Brown.

Hill, A. B. (1965). The environment and disease: Association or causation? *Proceedings of the Royal Society of Medicine, 58*, 295–300.

Kagan, A., Kannel, W. B., Dawber, T. R., & Revotskie, N. (1963). The coronary profile. *Annals of the New York Academy of Sciences, 97*, 883–894.

Kannel, W. B. (1979). Possible hazards of oral contraceptive use. *Circulation, 60*(3), 490–491.

Kannel, W. B., & Ellison, R. C. (1996). Alcohol and coronary heart disease: The evidence for a protective effect. *Clinica Chimica Acta; International Journal of Clinical Chemistry, 246*(1–2), 59–76.

Kannel, W. B., & McGee, D. L. (1979). Diabetes and cardiovascular disease. The Framingham study. *The Journal of the American Medical Association, 241*(19), 2035–2038.

Murray, J., & Ryan-Krause, P. (2010). Obesity in children with Down syndrome: Background and recommendations for management. *Pediatric Nursing, 36*(6), 314–319.

Ogden, C. L., Carroll, M. D., Curtin, L. R., Lamb, M. M., & Flegal, K. M. (2010). Prevalence of high body mass index in US children and adolescents, 2007–2008. *The Journal of the American Medical Association, 303*(3), 242–249.

Oleckno, W. A. (2002). *Essential epidemiology: Principles and applications.* Prospect Heights, IL: Waveland.

Pan, W., & Bai, H. (2009). A multivariate approach to a meta-analytic review of the effectiveness of the D.A.R.E. program. *International Journal of Environmental Research and Public Health, 6*(1), 267–277.

Reeder, B. A., Chen, Y., Macdonald, S. M., Angel, A., & Sweet, L. (1997). Regional and rural-urban differences in obesity in Canada. Canadian heart health surveys research group. *Canadian Medical Association Journal (Journal De l'Association Medicale Canadienne), 157*(Suppl 1), S10–16.

Rimmer, J. H., Yamaki, K., Lowry, B. M., Wang, E., & Vogel, L. C. (2010). Obesity and obesity-related secondary conditions in adolescents with intellectual/developmental disabilities. *Journal of Intellectual Disability Research, 54*(9), 787–794.

Ringwalt, C., Ennett, S. T., & Holt, K. D. (1991). An outcome evaluation of Project DARE (Drug Abuse Resistance Education). *Health Education Research, 6*, 327–337.

Rothman, K. J. (1986). *Modern epidemiology.* Boston: Little, Brown.

Soskolne, C. L., Jhangri, G. S., Scott, H. M., Brenner, D. R., Siemiatycki, J., Lakhani, R., et al. (2011). A population-based case-control study of occupational exposure to acids and the risk of lung cancer: Evidence for specificity of association. *International Journal of Occupational and Environmental Health, 17*(1), 1–8.

Susser, M. (1977). Judgement and causal inference: Criteria in epidemiologic studies. *American Journal of Epidemiology, 105*(1), 1–15.

Sutton, A. J., Jones, D. R., Abrams, K. R., Sheldon, T. A., & Song, F. (1999). Systematic reviews and meta-analysis: A structured review of the methodological literature. *Journal of Health Services Research & Policy, 4*(1), 49–55.

U.S. Public Health Service. Surgeon General's Advisory Committee on Smoking and Health. (1964). *Smoking and health; report of the advisory committee to the surgeon general of the public health service.* Washington, DC: Government Printing Office

Vincus, A. A., Ringwalt, C., Harris, M. S., & Shamblen, S. R. (2010). A short-term, quasi-experimental evaluation of D.A.R.E.'s revised elementary school curriculum. *Journal of Drug Education, 40*(1), 37–49.

West, S. L., & O'Neal, K. K. (2004). Project D.A.R.E. outcome effectiveness revisited. *American Journal of Public Health, 94*(6), 1027–1029.

Wolf, P. A., Dawber, T. R., Thomas, H. E., Jr., & Kannel, W. B. (1978). Epidemiologic assessment of chronic atrial fibrillation and risk of stroke: The Framingham study. *Neurology, 28*(10), 973–977.

Woods, J. L., Iuliano-Burns, S., & Walker, K. Z. (2011). Weight loss in elderly women in low-level care and its association with transfer to high-level care and mortality. *Clinical Interventions in Aging, 6*, 311–317.

Overview of Epidemiologic Study Designs

Goldilocks lay down in the first bed, but it was too hard. Then she lay down in the second bed, but it was too soft. Then she lay down in the third bed, and it was just right.

INTRODUCTION

Like Goldilocks in the children's story, *Goldilocks and the Three Bears*, researchers must choose a study design that best "fits" their research question. The carefully crafted research question must guide every element of the study—from overall design, to measurement, to analysis. In this chapter, we will consider the research questions of other investigators and see how the questions "fit" the study designs.

We assume that readers of this text are familiar with the taxonomy of epidemiologic research designs (case studies, cohort studies, randomized controlled trials, and so on). Instead of an exhaustive treatment of the details of these study designs, we present the designs in the context of their essential elements.[*]

ELEMENTS OF A STUDY DESIGN (HUIT)

The elements of epidemiologic research studies can be organized according to the acronym HUIT: **H**ypothesis tested or not; **U**nit of observation or analysis; **I**ntervention implemented or not; **T**iming of the measurement of exposure and outcome. The acronym is useful as a heuristic device for organizing study designs according to these elements.

Hypothesis

The research hypothesis is the statement of the association, causal relationship, or intervention effect we wish to test in our study of health phenomena. For example:

> "Rural residents of Western Canada are more likely to be obese compared to their urban counterparts."
>
> "The risk of lung cancer increases with the number of cigarettes smoked per day."
>
> "Students who participate in DARE are less likely to initiate drug use compared to students who do not participate in DARE."

Analytic studies, by definition, test hypotheses about the correlates, causes, or deterrents of morbidity and mortality.

In contrast, descriptive studies do not test hypotheses. Instead, they describe the distribution of a health phenomenon in terms of who has it, where it occurs, and when it begins and ends. The goal of this type of research is to answer general questions rather than test specific hypotheses. For example:

---

[*]For a review of the more specific details of epidemiologic study designs, see *Epidemiology for Public Health Practice* by Robert Friis and Thomas Sellers (2009).

"Is there a difference in the rates of CVD for men and women?"

"What is the prevalence of obesity among teens with Down syndrome?"

"What are the sociodemographic characteristics of Patient X with these unusual symptoms?"

Descriptive studies, by definition, do not test hypotheses.

Unit of Observation

The unit of observation is the single entity from which we collect our data. In epidemiologic research, the unit is either an individual person or a group. For the person unit, we collect and analyze individual data points, such as body mass index (BMI), marital status, experimental or control assignment, and so on. For the group unit, we consider the group as a single entity and collect and analyze average data such as per capita fat consumption, mean BMI, traffic deaths per 1,000 population, and so on.

Care should be taken in interpreting the results of studies using the group as the unit of analysis. An error or fallacy is made when the results of a group study are interpreted or applied to the situation of the individual. This error in interpretation is called the ecologic fallacy. The term for this error was coined in response to a study of suicide conducted by French social thinker Emile Durkheim in the 19th century. Durkheim compared the country-wide suicide rates for European countries that were predominantly Catholic or Protestant. He noted higher suicide rates for Protestant than for Catholic countries and concluded that something about the Catholic religion protects its followers from committing suicide (Durkheim, 1897). The problem with this conclusion is that Durkheim was unable to determine if the individuals who committed suicide were, in fact, Protestant. Perhaps, some or many of the people who committed suicide in the Protestant countries were, in fact, Catholic, or even Jewish or Muslim. This error is a classic example of the ecologic fallacy. Durkheim drew conclusions about relationships for individual persons based on results from group-level or average data.

The typical unit of analysis in epidemiologic studies is the individual person. However, two study designs (discussed in the next section) do utilize the group as the unit of observation.

Intervention

In epidemiologic research, an intervention is an effort implemented to prevent or improve the natural history of a disease or health problem. The effort can take the form of an experimental drug or surgical procedure, a health promotion campaign, a law, a screening program, a rehabilitation regimen, and so on. Evaluation studies determine the efficacy (success) of the intervention in preventing or treating the health problem.

In a true experimental design, the investigator manipulates the intervention by determining the inclusion or exclusion criteria of subjects included in the evaluation, who is in the experimental or control group, the dose or intensity of the intervention, the nature and design of the intervention and the placebo, the length of the follow-up period, and so on. Studies can also observe and measure the efficacy of interventions that are not manipulated by the intervention. The interventions are manipulated naturally, and this type of evaluation is called a natural experiment. The classic studies of the source of cholera outbreaks conducted by John Snow in 19th-century London are examples of natural experiments. What he was able to compare but not manipulate was the source of the water supply for those with and without cholera. Contemporary examples of natural experiments include the effect of fluoridating drinking water on the incidence and prevalence of dental caries, the impact of seat belt laws on traffic fatalities, and the influence of tobacco tax increases on the incidence of cigarette smoking.

Timing of the Exposure and Outcome

This element of the study design concerns itself with the timing of the measurement of the exposure thought to be related to the disease or outcome relative to the timing of the outcome measurement. In the natural course of disease onset, the exposure is measured at a point before the outcome measurement. However, under some conditions, it is necessary to measure the exposure and outcome at the same point in time or to measure the outcome at the beginning of the study and go back in time through the subjects' memories or through historical data, such as medical records and occupational exposures, to measure the exposure. Designs dependent on different configurations of this element are discussed in the following section.

TREATMENT OF HUIT ELEMENTS
IN STUDY DESIGNS

Table 3–1 presents epidemiologic study designs ordered from least to most rigorous in the context of the HUIT elements as well as the type of research goal they can address.

Table 3–2 shows the strengths and weaknesses of each class of designs.

Table 3–1 Study Designs by Research Goal and HUIT Elements

Research Goal	Study Design	Hypothesis Yes	Hypothesis No	Unit of Analysis Individual	Unit of Analysis Group	Intervention Yes	Intervention No	Timing of Measurement E O ⇒	Timing of Measurement E O ↻	Timing of Measurement E O ⇐
Descriptive/ association	Case report		•	•			•	•		
	Case series		•	•			•	•		
	Ecological	•			•		•	•	•	•
	Cross-sectional	•		•			•		•	
Causal	Case-control	•		•			•			•
	Retrospective cohort	•		•			•			•
	Prospective cohort	•		•			•	•		
	Ambispective cohort	•		•			•	•		•
Causal/ evaluation	Community trial	•			•	•		•		
	Randomized controlled trial	•		•		•		•		

E = exposure; O = outcome

Case Report and Case Series

A case report is the most basic descriptive design. Usually conducted in a clinical setting, it involves the description of symptoms and other potentially relevant characteristics for a single individual or patient. Case reports are used to gather and report information suggestive of potential hypotheses to be tested in more rigorous study designs. They are particularly important for examining emerging or rare health phenomena. Potential responsible exposures may emerge from the description of symptoms and sociodemographic, lifestyle, and other characteristics.

A case series is a collection of case reports describing the characteristics of a small number of individuals with similar symptoms. This design is slightly stronger than a case report because patterns of symptoms and characteristics begin to emerge when a number of patients are compared in an attempt to find similarities and differences. However, the number of individuals included in these studies is relatively small (typically less than 10) and insufficient to test hypotheses. Again, hypotheses can emerge from these studies.

The main disadvantages of case reports and series are the lack of a control or comparison group and the inability to address specific research questions.

Table 3–2 Strengths and Weaknesses of Study Designs

Study Design	Strengths	Weaknesses
Case report/case series	Identify new diseases	No control group
	Easy to conduct	Cannot answer specific research questions
	Generate hypotheses	
Ecological	Advantage of secondary data sources	Ecologic fallacy
	Easy to conduct	Imprecision in measure of exposure and outcome
	Ability to consider relevant social/community/group factors	
Cross-sectional	Can estimate prevalence	Not possible to examine temporal relationships between exposure and outcome
	Easy to conduct	
	Typically ethical	
	Efficient for including large numbers of subjects	Cannot estimate incidence
		Difficult to examine rare outcomes
Case-control	Efficient for rare outcomes and new diseases	Cannot estimate prevalence or incidence
		Uncertainty in temporal relationships
		Unknown external validity
		Potential for misclassification bias in terms of true cases and true controls
Cohort	Can estimate incidence	Expensive and time-intensive
	Can address temporal order of exposure and outcome	Inefficient for rare outcomes and those with long latency periods
	Efficient for rare exposures	
		Subject to nonresponse and attrition bias
		Potential for confounding
Experimental trials	Potential to minimize bias and confounding	Potential threat to external validity
	Ability to manipulate exposure	Ethical issues
	Best design to test causal relationships	Expensive and time-intensive
	Can establish temporal order of exposure and outcome	Dependence on subject retention

Common characteristics of cases can be observed, but without a comparison group it is not possible to demonstrate that these characteristics are specific to the cases and the outcome of interest. The discovery of common characteristics suggests the design of more rigorous studies with control groups to determine the specificity of these characteristics, which further suggests studies to examine potential causality.

Example: HIV/AIDS Case Study and Series

More than 30 years ago, on June 5, 1981, the Centers for Disease Control and Prevention (CDC), in its *Morbidity and Mortality Weekly Report*, described a higher than expected incidence of *Pneumocystis carinii* pneumonia (PCP) among otherwise healthy young men in Los Angeles, California (CDC, 1981). The number of cases of PCP was alarming because, previous to this report, PCP was seen rarely and only in patients with immune systems weakened by medical treatments, such as chemotherapy and organ transplantation. These young men were healthy, but had one characteristic in common—they were men who had sex with men (MSM). At this point, CDC investigators speculated that these men's case histories indicated that PCP was the result of a "disease acquired through sexual contact."

On July 8, 1982, CDC's *AIDS Surveillance Report* characterized cases of PCP and other opportunistic infections according to age, sex, race/ethnicity, sexual orientation, and residence (CDC, 1982). By December 22, 1983, surveillance reports added intravenous drug user, Haitian, and hemophiliac to the list of relevant patient characteristics (CDC, 1983). By December 3, 1984, heterosexual contact, blood transfusion recipient, and child of a parent with AIDS were added to the list of patient characteristics or groups (CDC, 1984). As a result of these case series, the vehicle for transmission was hypothesized to be human body fluids. **Table 3–3** shows a summary of these reports.

Ecological Study Design

Ecological studies are descriptive studies with groups as the unit of observation. Groups can be households, neighborhoods, schools, hospitals, states, countries, regions, and so on. Outcomes and potential exposures typically are measured during the same period of time and are aggregate measures such as averages, group prevalence, and number per capita population. Because exposure and outcome are measured at the same time and inferences cannot be made on an individual level, evidence of causality cannot be tested. Ecological designs can, to a limited extent, measure the temporal order of exposure and outcome, but the lack of precision in average measures makes it difficult to conclude with relative certainty that the exposure preceded the outcome. Ecological studies are useful in that they can analyze the role of social factors (e.g., norms) that are additive,

Table 3–3 AIDS Weekly Surveillance Report Patient Groups, December 31, 1984

	Adult/Adolescent				Total	
	Males	(%)	Females	(%)	Cases	(%)
Homosexual or bisexual	5,541	(78)	-----	(--)	5,541	(73)
IV drug user	1,042	(15)	275	(55)	1,317	(17)
Haitian	221	(3)	42	(9)	263	(3)
Hemophilia	49	(1)	0	(0)	49	(1)
Heterosexual contact	5	(0)	54	(11)	59	(1)
Transfusion	49	(1)	41	(8)	90	(1)
Other	206	(3)	84	(17)	290	(4)
Total	7,113	(100)	964	(100)	7,609	(100)

	Pediatric				Total	
	Males	(%)	Females	(%)	Cases	(%)
Parent with or at risk for AIDS	34	(64)	30	(81)	64	(71)
Hemophilia	4	(8)	0	(0)	4	(4)
Transfusion	10	(19)	2	(5)	12	(13)
Other	5	(9)	5	(14)	10	(11)
Total	53	(100)	37	(100)	90	(100)

Source: Modified from the AIDS Weekly Surveillence Report Patient Groups (1984, December 31). Retrieved from http://www.cdc.gov/hiv/topics/surveillance/resources/reports/pdf/surveillance84.pdf.

multiplicative, synergistic, or interactive relationships of individual components. They may be greater than the sum of their parts. Like case reports and series, ecological studies can be useful for generating hypotheses that would be tested in more rigorous study designs. However, as mentioned earlier, the primary weakness of the ecological design is the ecologic fallacy of interpreting results at the group level to the individual level.

Example: HIV/AIDS Ecological Study

In the interest of explaining the heterogeneous distribution of HIV between and within continents, an ecological study compared the observed and expected prevalence of HIV based on racial/ethnic composition (Pepin, 2005). Thirty-four populations in the Americas (including the countries of Brazil, Honduras, and Guyana, as well as the ethnic groups of African Americans and African Canadians) were compared. The populations were characterized by their composition of immigrants from Africa, Europe, and Asia. Then, the prevalence of HIV in each population was predicted by the ethnic composition and prevalence of HIV in the mother countries. These expected prevalences were then compared to the observed prevalences, and a high level of agreement was found in most of the populations.

The investigator acknowledged that several confounders, such as sexual activity, and cofactors of transmission may explain these similarities, although it was not possible to measure these. He concluded that the relationships are too strong to be due to potential confounders and that biological susceptibility to HIV is the likely explanation for these results. This conclusion warrants further investigation. It is plausible, but this study on its own cannot support a causal relationship between genetic susceptibility and HIV prevalence.

Cross-Sectional Study Design

The unit of analysis for cross-sectional studies is the individual person. These studies are also called prevalence studies, because they allow the calculation of the prevalence of health phenomena in the study population. Examples include one-time surveys and biological tests. The defining characteristic of cross-sectional studies is that the exposure and outcome are measured at the same point in time. This design is equipped to identify factors that are associated with the health phenomena, but causality cannot be established without the proper temporal order of exposure first and outcome later. Correlates of the outcome can be interpreted as risk factors, but not as true causes. However, the identification of risk factors in cross-sectional studies suggests causal factors to be examined in etiologic studies.

Cross-sectional studies are relatively inexpensive and efficient for including potentially large numbers of subjects. They are also ethical in terms of typically involving minimal risk to subjects. However, they are relatively inefficient for studying rare diseases in that extremely large samples would be required to capture enough cases to support analysis.

Example: HIV Cross-Sectional Study

We travel to Madrid, Spain, for a cross-sectional study of injection drug users (IDU) (Bravo Portela, Barrio Anta, de la Fuente de Hoz, et al., 1996). Structured interviews of 441 current IDUs measured awareness of their HIV status, drug use, and sexual behaviors in the month prior to the interview. Of those who knew their HIV status, 48.6% were positive. The results of the study showed multiple correlations between various HIV risk behaviors and awareness of HIV status. Risk behaviors included passing and taking used syringes, unprotected sexual activity with different types of sexual partners, types of drugs used, and history of incarceration. There was no clear outcome in this study because associations between confirmed HIV status (the logical outcome) and risk factors were not reported. Instead, the value of this study, as in cross-sectional studies generally, is the reporting of relevant prevalences. The prevalence of self-reported HIV infection was very high in this sample, as were HIV risk behaviors, including sharing syringes (21.7%) and not always using condoms (67.5%).

Case-Control Study Design

The unit of analysis in case-control studies is the individual. The study uses true exposure and outcome measures that are anchored in measured time. The study begins with the outcome measure and relies on participants' memories or medical records to go back in time to measure the potential exposure. A unique feature of this design is that individuals with the outcome of interest (cases) are compared to individuals who do not have the outcome but were at risk for it (controls) to determine differences in past exposure to the potential cause of the health phenomena. Another unique feature of this design is that only one measure of association between exposure and outcome is appropriate—the odds ratio.

Case-control studies are especially valuable for studying rare or emerging disorders. Selecting cases first is an efficient and relatively inexpensive approach for these types of health phenomena. However, care should be taken in defining and selecting both cases and controls. The selection of cases involves two tasks: (1) defining a case conceptually, and (2) identifying a case operationally (Lasky & Stolley, 1994). The conceptual definition should be neither too broad nor too exclusive. A case definition that is too broad will likely include subjects who are not true cases, resulting in misclassification bias and artificially weakening the relationship between exposure and outcome. A definition that is too exclusive would likely lead to difficulty identifying cases and unnecessarily increasing study costs. However, the balance between inclusivity and exclusivity should weigh toward exclusivity, because misclassification bias would seriously compromise the validity of study results.

Cases and controls are identified from either clinical or general population sources. Clinical sources like hospitals or medical practices are efficient for disorders that sometimes require treatment and rehabilitation. However, cases found in clinical settings usually represent the most severe manifestation of the disorder. If a clinical source for cases is used, then the same clinical source should be used to identify controls. For example, if cases of lung cancer are selected from Hospital A, controls treated in Hospital A for illnesses other than lung cancer should be chosen. However, patients with illnesses too similar to lung cancer, such as emphysema, should be avoided as controls due to similar disease etiology.

Cases can also be found in nonclinical settings through disease registries, other studies (cross-sectional or cohort), and even advertisements. For these cases, controls should be chosen from the same neighborhood, community, or region. Friends, relatives, and coworkers of cases can also be used as controls. Whenever possible and practical, controls should be similar to cases in important outcome-relevant characteristics, such as age, gender, occupation, medical history, residence, and so on.

A potential weakness of case-control studies is an inability to calculate incidence or prevalence of the outcome. Incidence is impossible to measure because the study travels back in time so cases cannot be measured as they emerge. Prevalence cannot be measured because the relative distribution of cases and controls is artificial, having been predetermined by the investigator. The investigator may need 50% of her sample to have the outcome to support the planned analysis, whereas the true prevalence of the outcome in the general populations is only 5%. Similarly, the extent to which the sample represents the population of individuals with the outcome (external validity) cannot be established because the sample was purposively selected to include a large proportion of cases. Another weakness of the case-control design is uncertainty about the true temporal order of exposure and outcome due to potential weaknesses of available historical data. The exposure measure is only as valid as the quality of data collected by someone other than the investigator or the memories of the study subjects. Attempts should be made to evaluate the quality of this data.

Example: HIV Case-Control Study

After observing that the majority of HIV cases in Belgium were among Europeans who spent significant amounts of time living in Africa, a case-control study was designed to determine the responsible risk behaviors (Bonneux, Van der Stuyft, Taelman, et al., 1988). From a group of male Belgian advisers and expatriates living in Africa, 33 men with HIV were chosen as cases, and 119 men without HIV were selected as controls. Cases and controls were interviewed to determine their past risk behaviors while residing in Africa. Calculated odds ratios indicated the odds of having had sexual contact with local women were 14.7 times greater for HIV-positive men compared to HIV-negative men; 10.8 times greater for having had sexual contact with prostitutes; and 13.5 greater for having had medically prescribed injections by unqualified medical staff. This study, conducted early in the history of AIDS (1988), was one of the first to show that heterosexual contact is a viable mechanism for the transmission of HIV.

Cohort Studies

Cohort studies, also called incidence studies, are designed to measure the exposure and outcome in the context of time. In this design, individual subjects are followed over time to measure the exposure when it happens (in real time or historically), then measure the outcome at a point in time after the exposure. Because the outcome is measured exactly or approximately when it happens, the incidence of the health phenomena (new cases) can be determined in cohort studies. The strength of this design is the ability to demonstrate the temporal order of the exposure and outcome—a necessary criteria to determine causality.

While case-control studies are limited to odds ratios for measuring associations between exposures and outcomes, cohort studies allow the use of risk differences, risk ratios, and odds ratios for evaluating associations. The concept of "risk" is meaningful because the outcome or disorder is measured as incidence. Both risk and incidence are time-dependent.

Cohort studies can be prospective, retrospective, or ambispective. These designs are illustrated in **Figure 3–1**. Prospective cohort designs move forward in time. They first measure the exposure, then the outcome or disorder. Both exposure and outcome are measured directly in real time. This design allows the most flexibility in terms of exposure measures. Surveys, medical tests, and observations can all be accomplished in prospective designs.

Retrospective cohort designs move backward in study time. The outcome is measured at the start of the study, and the exposure, which actually occurred before the start of the study, is determined by historical data such as medical records, employment histories, and subjects' memories. Exposure measures are limited by what data are available, but this weakness is balanced by the savings in the costs of measuring them in real time and the significant benefit of efficiently measuring rare outcomes. Subjects at high risk for the outcome are chosen for the study, so fewer numbers of subjects are needed to achieve sufficient numbers with the outcome. The retrospective cohort design differs from the case-control design in that the former design chooses subjects at risk for the outcome, naturally including those with and without the outcome; and the latter purposely chooses those with the outcome, then a group of controls without the disorder. In this regard, the prevalence of the outcome is manipulated and not natural.

Ambispective cohort designs move both forward and backward in time. With this design, the exposure is measured twice—historically and in real time during

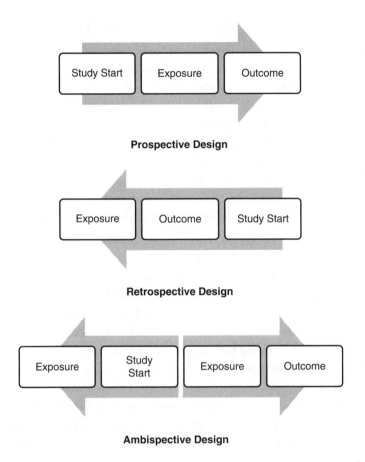

FIGURE 3–1 Cohort Study Designs

the study period. The design allows a more precise measure of exposures in terms of time. It can be determined if the exposure is longer or shorter term or variable in terms of coming and going. For example, a study about hip replacement (outcome in the future) can start with adults aged 20 to 40 years and measure their current and future physical activity (contemporary exposure) as well as school and other historical records to determine their childhood experience with organized sports—type, intensity, and duration.

The main disadvantage of cohort studies is that they tend to be very expensive and time-intensive. The study is weakened substantially with high attrition (i.e., more than 20%) of subjects between measurement points (baseline to subsequent follow-ups). Considerable resources and staff time are typically needed to maximize retention rates and, subsequently, the validity of the study sample. The design is also inefficient for rare outcomes and those with a very long latency period (time from exposure to outcome). Retrospective cohorts are often utilized to address this inefficiency. On the other hand, cohort studies can be efficient for studying rare exposures in that cohorts can be selected based on their likelihood of exposure (e.g., occupation groups, residents of high-risk areas). Finally, confounding can be a particular problem for cohort studies in that a strong design would anticipate and measure potential confounders from the start of the study. This is not often the case, so appropriate measures are not available to test confounding, and subjects have not been matched on confounding characteristics to minimize their effect on the relationship between exposure and outcome.

Example: HIV Cohort Studies

Thirty years into the AIDS epidemic, it is accepted and common knowledge that male homosexual activity is an effective vehicle for HIV infection. However, in 1984, this route of transmission was suspected, but not proven. Hence, a cohort of 66 homosexual men was followed from 1982 to 1983 (Goedert, Sarngadharan, Biggar, et al., 1984). During this period, the seroconversion (infection) rate was 1.2% per month. Exposures strongly associated with seroconversion were large numbers of homosexual partners and receptive anal intercourse. Perhaps more informative, there was an interaction between number of partners and receptive intercourse in the form of a dose-response relationship—the greater the number of partners and incidents of receptive intercourse, the greater the risk of seroconversion.

A retrospective cohort study of gay men in San Francisco examined the association between drug and alcohol use and risky sexual activity for AIDS (Stall, McKusick, Wiley, et al., 1986). Men who in 1985 abstained from combining substance use and sexual activity were unlikely to have engaged in risky sexual activity (i.e., unprotected sex) during the prior year. The investigators conclude that combining substance use and sexual activity puts one at risk for unsafe sex practices. Although the relationship is plausible, this study design was unable to prove that the risky sex and the substance use occurred during the same event.

Experimental Trials

Experimental study designs are the gold standard of designs. In fact, Sir Austin Bradford Hill included experimental verification of results as a criterion to establish causality. Experimental studies, particularly randomized controlled trials, are the most rigorous because of their use of random assignment to exposure groups, which helps control classification bias and confounding (both discussed later). The ideal experimental design includes the following elements:

1. A pretest measurement of the outcome,
2. Random assignment of subjects into at least two groups—experimental and control,
3. Careful monitoring of the delivery of the exposure, and
4. Posttest measurement of the outcome.

The pretest, exposure, then posttest design follows the proper temporal ordering of exposure and outcome. This is the necessary criteria to establish that the exposure causes the outcome. The pre- and posttest measures allow the direct examination of change as a result of the exposure.

Comparing measures of change for experimental and control groups can indicate if any change during the study period is, in fact, the result of the exposure. If there is a significant difference in change between groups, then the causal mechanism can be attributed to the exposure. Random assignment of subjects into experimental or control groups means that each subject has the same probability of being assigned to one or the other group. An unequal probability of assignment could result in classification bias where one group is systematically different from the other. This difference could distort the association between exposure and outcome by either artificially inflating or deflating the relationship. The result is a biased or incorrect study result if this difference is not an intended aspect of the study design. Sometimes random assignment into groups is not possible, practical, or even ethical. Without random assignment to exposure groups, the study design is called quasi-experimental. This design is weaker than a true experiment with random assignment to the exposure.

Careful monitoring of the delivery of the exposure is another way to prevent or minimize bias between groups. The goal is to avoid cross-contamination where control subjects experience some aspect of the exposure, and experimental subjects miss some or all of the exposure. Cross-contamination would artificially deflate the strength of the association between exposure and outcome. If it does occur, even with careful monitoring, investigators can decide to include subjects originally assigned to the experimental group but who did not get the full dose of the exposure in the experimental group, called intention to treat, or can decide to move them into the control group, called per protocol. Again, the goal is to try to minimize bias between groups.

Experiment and Evaluation

Evaluation studies typically utilize the experimental design, but the purpose of the evaluation is different from the classic experimental study. The purpose of the latter is to provide support that an exposure causes an outcome. The goal of evaluation studies, on the other hand, is to determine if an intervention (e.g., medical treatment, drug, program, or campaign) is effective in preventing or minimizing the outcome or disorder. The targeted outcome of the intervention is called the experimental endpoint. Interventions that prevent the outcome are called prophylactic. Those that minimize or prevent escalation of the outcome are called therapeutic.

The unit of analysis for evaluation studies can be either the individual or a group, such as a school, neighborhood, community, or state. Evaluations of groups are called community trials. As in ecologic studies, outcome measures are group averages (e.g., group prevalence, means, per capita measures). The ecologic fallacy can be an issue in community trials if group results are interpreted on the individual level. Evaluations of individuals are called clinical trials or randomized controlled trials.

Ideally, random assignment to experimental and control groups is used no matter the unit of analysis. However, random assignment can be difficult in community trials because of practical and political reasons. Only when randomization is used in evaluations of individuals can the study be called a randomized controlled trial. This is the strongest design in terms of minimizing bias between exposure groups. To further strengthen the study, blinding is used. Blinding is preventing the knowledge of group assignment (experimental or control) among subjects. Double blinding is not allowing the investigator to know subject assignment. Blinding is intended to prevent bias in outcome assessments between groups.

Even though the experimental design, especially the randomized controlled trial, is considered the gold standard study design because of its ability to minimize bias and confounding, the design does have its disadvantages. The main disadvantages are the cost in resources and time, and the potential ethical issues. Ethical issues often arise when subjects are exposed (or not exposed) to a drug, therapy, program, or some other type of intervention. The potential harm involved in administering risky treatments and withholding effective treatments must be addressed and minimized. Because of this and other practical and ethical issues, another limitation of this study design is the potential threat to external validity of the study sample. Strict inclusionary and exclusionary criteria (e.g., minimum threshold of health status, absence of complicating conditions) may be necessary for ethical and practical reasons. Adherence to such criteria can limit the extent to which study subjects are representative of all individuals with or at risk for the outcome under study. Similarly, administration of the intervention typically requires a controlled setting to maximize the fidelity of its delivery—a setting that may be artificial compared to real-world conditions. Finally, as for cohort studies, retention of subjects is a major priority in experimental designs with posttest measurements. Poor retention weakens the generalizability of study results, and adequate retention typically requires large expenditures of resources.

Example: Population-Based Interventions for Reducing HIV

A review of randomized controlled trials for HIV and sexually transmitted infection (STI) prevention found that such interventions are generally ineffective (Wilkinson & Rutherford, 2001). Published studies of the results of randomized controlled trials in which the unit of analysis was either a community or treatment facility were selected for the review. Appropriate randomization methods, blinding, and patient attrition were evaluated as inclusion criteria. Communities or treatment facilities were randomly assigned to either experimental or control conditions. Five behavioral intervention trials were selected. Outcomes or endpoints of the trials included incident HIV infection, frequency of STIs, condom use, and quality of HIV/STI treatment. Modest increases in condom use with casual partners and quality of treatment were found, but the interventions resulted in very little or no reductions in HIV and STI incidence and prevalence.

Hybrid Study Designs

Epidemiologic studies also combine two or more study designs into hybrids—combining parts or the whole of each design. A common hybrid design is the nested case-control study. Generally, the term *nested* refers to something that occupies or resides in something else. In the context of study designs, a nested design is one in which a particular type of study emerges from an earlier study of a different design. Often, case-control studies develop from cohort studies. In the conduct of the cohort study, cases and controls are identified (based on the incidence of the outcome) and analyzed in an additional case-control study. In this common example, the case-control study is nested in the cohort study.

Another type of hybrid study is the combined analysis of group- and individual-level data. This particular type of hybrid study is called the multilevel design. The advantages of this design are the avoidance of the ecologic fallacy by analyzing individual-level data and the consideration of potentially important group-level factors such as laws, norms, resources, physical environment, and so on. An additional advantage is the low cost of analyzing group-level data that is often collected by other investigators. As this type of hybrid design has grown in popularity, multilevel analytic techniques have also developed.

Example: HIV Multilevel Study

Group- and individual-level data were analyzed to test the hypothesis that societal conditions influence high-risk sexual behaviors in Africa (Uchudi, Magadi, & Mostazir, 2011). Individual-level data measured sexual behaviors, and group-level data measured community norms and social change. The study showed that individuals living in communities with permissive sexual norms and tolerance of polygamy were more likely than others to have multiple sex partners. In addition, those with multiple partners were more likely than others to live in communities experiencing rapid social change in the form of education, urbanization, and work for cash.

CONCLUSION

In the real world of research, investigators rarely, if ever, have access to enough resources of time, money, and staff to implement the ideal study design to address their research questions. The research question should be the driving force of the study design. However, without appropriate resources, the question may need to be limited or altered so that a practical operationalizable study can be conducted to address the research question with appropriate validity, precision, and other forms of methodological rigor. An alteration of the question may result in and be a result of a modification of the research design. This interrelationship between research question and design is illustrated in **Figure 3–2**.

Thinking of the research design as a fulcrum balancing a scale, the shape and placement of the study design must balance the available study resources and the acceptable level of methodological rigor. The two-sided arrow connecting the study question and design illustrates the interaction and necessary adjustment in both the question and design in the interest of balancing resources and rigor. A researcher's ability to achieve this balance in the process of formulating the research question and designing the study decidedly improves with experience. Inexperienced researchers tend to aim too high in formulating a research question that is too broad or virtually impossible and/or impractical to operationalize. Sage advice for the novice researcher is to seek the guidance of a seasoned researcher in this initial process.

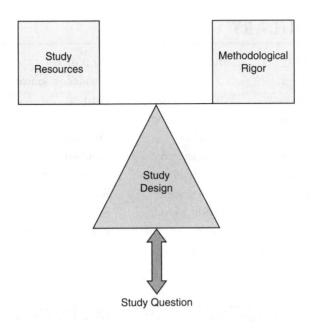

FIGURE 3–2 Relationship Between Study Design, Resources, and Methodological Rigor

Assuming the availability of adequate resources, the following are examples of specific research questions and their appropriate study designs:

Question: What is the prevalence of malignant meningiomas among adults in upstate New York?

Design: Cross-sectional study (no exposure studied; prevalence at one point in time).

Question: Is cell phone use related to incident malignant meningiomas?

Design: Retrospective cohort or case-control study (outcome is rare and takes years to develop).

Question: Do laws forbidding cell phone use while driving in New York state result in a decrease in malignant meningiomas?

Design: Ecologic study (compare incidence of tumors before and after implementation of the law).

Question: Does drug X slow the rate of growth of malignant meningiomas?

Design: Randomized controlled trial (with ethical consideration of appropriate treatment for the control group).

VOCABULARY

Ambispective	Double blinding	Per protocol
Blinding	Ecologic study	Population source
Case-control study	Ecologic fallacy	Posttest
Case series study	Experimental study	Pretest
Case study	Evaluation	Prospective
Classification bias	Gold standard	Randomization
Clinical source	Group-level	Randomized controlled trial
Cohort study	Hybrid designs	Retrospective
Community trial	Individual-level	Selection bias
Control group	Intention to treat	Unit of observation
Cross-sectional study	Multilevel study	

STUDY QUESTIONS AND EXERCISES

1. You finally receive funding to study the potential risk factors for an extremely rare blood disorder.
   a. What study design would be most appropriate for this research?
   b. Justify the choice of design.
   c. What are the strengths and limitations of this design?
2. Describe your hypothetical study of the blood disorder from problem 1.
   a. What are the characteristics of the subjects you would select for the study?
   b. What exposures, outcomes, and potential confounders would you measure?
   c. What would be the focus of your analysis?
3. You hypothesize that women are more vulnerable to depression than are men.
   a. What study design would you use to test this hypothesis?
   b. Justify the choice of design.
   c. What are the strengths and limitations of this design?
4. Describe your hypothetical study of gender and depression from problem 3.
   a. What are the characteristics of the subjects you would select for the study?

  b. What exposures, outcomes, and potential confounders would you measure?

  c. What would be the focus of your analysis?

5. You want to determine the risk factors for autism.

  a. What study design would you use to test this hypothesis?

  b. Justify the choice of design.

  c. What are the strengths and limitations of this design?

6. Describe your hypothetical study of the risk factors for autism from problem 5.

  a. What are the characteristics of the subjects you would select for the study?

  b. What exposures, outcomes, and potential confounders would you measure?

  c. What would be the focus of your analysis?

7. Describe a community trial to test the efficacy of a weight-loss program.

  a. What are the characteristics of the communities you would choose for the study?

  b. What exposures, outcomes, and potential confounders would you measure?

  c. What would be the focus of your analysis?

  d. What are the strengths and limitations of this design?

8. Describe a randomized controlled trial to test the efficacy of a smoking cessation program.

  a. What are the characteristics of the subjects you would choose for the study?

  b. What exposures, outcomes, and potential confounders would you measure?

  c. What would be the focus of your analysis?

  d. What are the strengths and limitations of this design?

9. Consider your particular research interest and focus.

  a. What study design(s) would you use to address this research interest?

  b. Justify the choice of design(s).

10. Outline your study in terms of the key elements of the design.

11. Evaluate the feasibility of your study design.

  a. What factors might facilitate the success of the study?

  b. What factors might impede the success of the study?

  c. How might you overcome these impediments?

REFERENCES

Bonneux, L., Van der Stuyft, P., Taelman, H., Cornet, P., Goilav, C., van der Groen, G., et al. (1988). Risk factors for infection with human immunodeficiency virus among European expatriates in Africa. *BMJ (Clinical Research Ed.), 297*(6648), 581–584.

Bravo Portela, M. J., Barrio Anta, G., de la Fuente de Hoz, L., Colomo Gomez, C., Royuela Morales, L., & Estebanez Estebanez, P. (1996). Risk behaviors for HIV transmission among the recent clients of a syringe-exchange program in madrid, 1993. [Conductas de riesgo para transmision del VIH entre los usuarios recientes de un programa de intercambio de jeringas en Madrid, 1993] *Gaceta Sanitaria/S.E.S.P.A.S, 10*(57), 261–273.

Centers for Disease Control and Prevention. (1981). *Pneumocystis* pneumonia—Los Angeles. *Morbidity and Mortality Weekly Report, 30*(21), 1–3.

Centers for Disease Control and Prevention. (1982). Kaposi's sarcoma (KS), pneumocystis carinii pneumonia (PCP), and other opportunistic infections (OI): Cases reported to CDC as of July 8, 1982. *Morbidity and Mortality Weekly Report, 31*(26), 353–354, 360–361.

Centers for Disease Control and Prevention. AIDS Activity. (1983). Acquired immunodeficiency syndrome (AIDS). *Weeky Surveillance Report—United States.*

Centers for Disease Control and Prevention. AIDS Activity. (1984). Acquired immunodeficiency syndrome (AIDS). *Weekly Surveillance Report—United States.*

Durkheim, E. (1897). *Le suicide; étude de sociologie.* Paris: F. Alcan.

Friis, R. H., & Sellers, T. A. (2009). *Epidemiology for public health practice* (4th ed.). Sudbury, MA: Jones and Bartlett Publishers.

Goedert, J. J., Sarngadharan, M. G., Biggar, R. J., Weiss, S. H., Winn, D. M., Grossman, R. J., et al. (1984). Determinants of retrovirus (HTLV-III) antibody and immunodeficiency conditions in homosexual men. *Lancet, 2*(8405), 711–716.

Lasky, T., & Stolley, P. D. (1994). Selection of cases and controls. *Epidemiologic Reviews, 16*(1), 6–17.

Pepin, J. (2005). From the old world to the new world: An ecologic study of population susceptibility to HIV infection. *Tropical Medicine & International Health: TM & IH, 10*(7), 627–639.

Stall, R., McKusick, L., Wiley, J., Coates, T. J., & Ostrow, D. G. (1986). Alcohol and drug use during sexual activity and compliance with safe sex guidelines for AIDS: The AIDS behavioral research project. *Health Education Quarterly, 13*(4), 359–371.

Uchudi, J., Magadi, M., & Mostazir, M. (2011). A multilevel analysis of the determinants of high-risk sexual behaviour in Sub-Saharan Africa. *Journal of Biosocial Science,* 1–23. Available on CJO 2011 doi:10.1017/S0021932011000654.

Wilkinson, D., & Rutherford, G. (2001). Population-based interventions for reducing sexually transmitted infections, including HIV infection. *Cochrane Database of Systematic Reviews (Online), 2*(2), CD001220.

CHAPTER 4

Research Ethics

LEARNING OBJECTIVES

By the end of this chapter the reader will be able to:
- Trace the history of human subjects protection.
- Utilize the components of current protection regulations.
- Adapt study procedures to the special needs of vulnerable populations.

CHAPTER OUTLINE

Two of the worst patients, with the tendons in the ham rigid (a symptom none the rest had) were put under a course of sea water. Of this they drank half a pint every day.

—James Lind, A Treatise of
the Scurvy, 1757

INTRODUCTION

A half a pint of sea water a day? James Lind, most noted for proving through an experimental study in 18th-century England that citric acid prevents scurvy, would have to demonstrate today that consuming sea water would not cause harm to his human subjects—12 sailors—before beginning his study. Providing benefit rather than harm, or beneficence, is one of the three central requirements for ethical research with human subjects. Consideration of potential harm to subjects involves a careful investigation, anticipation, and weighing of the risks and benefits of the study. A truly ethical study would have benefits that outweigh risks to subjects. In Lind's (1757) study, the sailors were already suffering from scurvy, and the benefit of proving that citrus fruit is a preventative did not outweigh the risks to the sailors from consuming sea water and being denied citrus fruit for the purposes of the study. Today, Lind's study protocol certainly would not meet the requirement of beneficence and would not be approved to proceed.

Subject autonomy is the second requirement for ethical research using human subjects. This requirement has two components: (1) respecting the decision-making capacity of persons and, when appropriate, (2) protecting individuals with diminished capacity for self-determination (National Commission for the Protection of Human Subjects of Biomedical and Behavioral Research [NCPHSBBR], 1979). Individuals who lack the maturity and/or physical, social, or mental capacity to make informed decisions require and deserve special protections to consent to and participate in research studies. There is no published report of a consent procedure for Lind's scurvy study, but it is unlikely that sailors confined to a ship at sea and suffering from scurvy have the appropriate autonomy to consent to research.

The third requirement is justice—the fair distribution of the burdens and benefits of research across groups of people. The clearest example of injustice is research that uses only disadvantaged persons as research subjects and makes the benefits of the research available to only advantaged individuals. A less clear but appropriate example is clinical trials using only men as subjects and marketing the tested drug to men and women. Due to biological and other differences, the drug may be unsafe or ineffective for women. Lind studied confined and somewhat incapacitated sailors to determine a prevention of scurvy that is available for those who can afford to buy it. Citrus fruit was not indigenous to 18th-century England, so such fruit was available only for purchase for those who could afford it.

HISTORICAL DEVELOPMENT OF HUMAN SUBJECTS PROTECTION IN RESEARCH

The requirements of beneficence, autonomy, and justice, as well as other regulations in research, were developed in response to historical flagrant abuses of human subjects. James Lind's 18th-century study forcing the consumption of sea water by sick and confined sailors is an early but comparatively mild example of research abuse. The 20th century witnessed both the abuses and the development of protective regulations.

Nazi Experiments and the Nuremberg Code

Although referred to as the Nazi "experiments," there was nothing scientific about the horrific events that occurred in European concentration camps during World War II (1939–1945). Led by Josef Mengele, a geneticist by training, "experiments" were conducted using camp prisoners, especially twin children, in an attempt to manipulate physical characteristics and test the effects of wartime conditions. These included injecting dye into children's eyes, sewing children together, freezing and depriving oxygen, unnecessary amputations, and "living" autopsies. If the experiments were not working properly or results were not interesting, Mengele would have the subjects killed. These were extreme examples of human subject abuses with no beneficence, respect, or justice.

These horrific events were revealed during the Nuremberg Trials for Nazi war crimes in 1946–1947. One significant outcome of the trials was the Nuremberg Code of 1947. These were the first formal directives for human experimentation. The purpose was to protect the rights and well-being of human subjects in research. The directives are presented in **Figure 4–1**. The foundations of beneficence and respect can be seen in these codes.

Tuskegee Syphilis Study and U.S. Protection Regulations

In 1932, the United States Public Health Service began a study called the "Tuskegee Study of Untreated Syphilis in the Negro Male." It turned into a 40-year study of the natural history of syphilis among 600 mostly poor and uneducated black men in Tuskegee, Alabama. Even with the general acceptance of penicillin as an effective treatment of syphilis in 1947, the men were not offered this treatment. Although the subjects freely agreed to be examined and treated with the ineffective methods of the 1930s, they were neither told of the

1. The voluntary consent of the human subject is absolutely necessary.

2. The experiment should yield fruitful results for the good of society, with no alternative method for obtaining these results.

3. The experiment should be based on the results of animal experiments and knowledge of the natural history of the problem under study.

4. The experiment should avoid all unnecessary physical and mental harm.

5. No experiment should be conducted that is known or suspected to cause disabling injury or death.

6. Risks of the experiment should never outweigh the benefits.

7. Proper precautions should be made to prevent injury, disability, and death.

8. The experiment should be conducted only by scientifically qualified persons.

9. Subjects should be free to withdraw from the study at any time.

10. The investigator must terminate the experiment if injury, disability, or death appears possible.

FIGURE 4–1 The Nuremberg Code (1947)

Source: U.S. Government Printing Office. (1949). *Trials of war criminals before the Nuremberg Military Tribunals under Control Council Law, 10*(2), 181–182. Washington, DC.

study and its real purpose, nor given the choice to quit the study and receive adequate treatment (Curran, 1973). Both autonomy and beneficence were violated, and injustice was also evident in the use of poor, uneducated, and racially disadvantaged subjects.

Astonishingly, the study continued until 1972, and was terminated only after its purpose and history were widely publicized. Most of the men had died of syphilis and other causes, and many of their wives and children were infected with syphilis. As a result of this horrific study, the National Research Act and 45 CFR 46 were signed into law in 1974 (Department of Health and Human Services [DHHS], 2009). Among other things, the act required researchers to obtain voluntary informed consent from subjects and established institutional review boards (IRBs) at universities and research facilities. The mandate of IRBs is to review study protocols and approve them only if they meet ethical standards of informed voluntary consent, and if the benefits are greater than the risks.

Additional Studies and Regulations

Two U.S. studies conducted in the 1950s and 1960s had tenuous violations of beneficence, but flagrant violations of autonomy and justice. The 1956 Willowbrook hepatitis study injected mentally disabled children at Willowbrook State School in New York with hepatitis A virus to study the immunity response in pursuit of an effective vaccine (Krugman, 1986). The benefit of a vaccine as well as immunity for the children is substantial. Parental consent was obtained. The risk of harm was minimized by the investigators' claim that most, if not all of the children will be exposed to the virus eventually at the school and that this controlled exposure will result in the most mild cases of hepatitis.

The study violated autonomy by using disabled children who cannot consent because of their immaturity and limited mental capacity, and by using arguably coercive consent procedures with their parents. Due to budget problems and other political issues at the school, there was only room in the hepatitis unit of the school for new students. Therefore, admission to the school required consent to the study. This requirement unethically blurs the boundary between practice and research.

The Willowbrook study also violated the issue of justice by choosing to study children at the school rather than adult teachers and staff who could also be exposed naturally to hepatitis A in the school. In addition, and arguably most importantly, the natural epidemic of hepatitis in the school could have been minimized, or even prevented, by eliminating the overcrowding and unsanitary conditions at the school. Instead, the investigators took advantage of these adverse conditions to conduct their study.

A second landmark unethical study was the 1963 NY Jewish Chronic Disease Hospital study (Katz, Capron, & Glass, 1972). This study's investigators injected 19 critically ill (from non-cancer diseases) patients with cancer cells to demonstrate natural immunity to cancer. None of the subjects developed cancer as a result of the study. Before the study began, investigators were satisfied that subjects were in no danger of developing cancer as a result of the injections. However, subject autonomy was compromised by the fact that the patients and their doctors were told that the subjects were being injected with cells, but not that they were cancer cells. Consent was verbal and decidedly not informed. Justice was also compromised by the fact that information gained from the study would not benefit the subjects who will likely perish as a result of their existing non-cancer diseases.

These studies illustrate human subject abuses that led to the creation and ongoing revision of ethical regulations for medical research involving human subjects. The 1964 World Medical Association (WMA) Declaration of Helsinki set forth ethical principles, many of which addressed the requirement of informed consent. The declaration was the first to suggest an independent committee to evaluate and monitor the ethical conduct of human subject research. It also expanded the notion of subject autonomy by formalizing what is and is not informed consent for persons who are and are not able to give such consent. Issues of potential conflicts of interest involving investigators were also introduced.

In 1979, regulations and ethical guidelines were established and are still used in research today (NCPHSBBR, 1979). The Belmont Report, named after the Belmont Conference Center in Elkridge, Maryland, where the committee meeting took place, was drafted and approved by the 11-member National Commission for the Protection of Human Subjects of Biomedical and Behavioral Research. The purpose of the report was to broaden and clarify the rules set forth in the Nuremberg Code, the Helsinki Declaration, and the 1974 federal regulations. The report has three parts—Part A: Boundaries Between Practice and Research, Part B: Basic Ethical Principles, and Part C: Applications. **Figure 4–2** presents more information about the three parts. The practical application of the three basic ethical principles (autonomy, beneficence, and justice) is the topic of the next section.

PRACTICAL APPLICATIONS OF CURRENT HUMAN SUBJECTS REGULATIONS

Once a study design is nearly finalized, it is time for the investigator to submit for review the study protocol, forms, and related materials to the IRB at his or her university or research facility. What follows is an example of the type of information typically required in the initial review form.

Boundary Between Practice and Research

- Purpose of medical practice is to provide diagnosis, preventive treatment, or therapy
- Purpose of research is to test a hypothesis, draw conclusions, and make generalizations
- Research and practice can be combined when research is designed to evaluate a therapy
- Treatment should not require research participation

Basic Ethical Principles

- Respect for persons (autonomy)—subjects should enter research voluntarily and with adequate information
- Beneficence—do not harm; maximize benefits and minimize possible risks
- Justice—classes of subjects should not, without scientific justification, be included or excluded from research; benefits from treatment should be made available to all who need it, including those who participated in the study

Applications

- Informed consent (autonomy)—complete disclosure of all aspects of the research; verified subject comprehension of research procedures; voluntary consent without coercion or undue influence
- Assessment of risks and benefits (benificence)—probabilities and magnitudes of possible harm and anticipated benefits; systematic, nonarbitrary analysis of risks and benefits should be conducted whenever possible
- Selection of subjects (justice)—individual justice means that benefical research should not include only advantaged persons and risky research should not include only disadvantaged persons; social justice means the order of classes of subjects selected should start with the most competent (mature and able) and move to the least capable (children, disabled, prisoners) only when scientifically justifiable

FIGURE 4–2 The Belmont Report (1979)

Source: United States National Commission for the Protection of Human Subjects of Biomedical and Behavioral Research. (1979). *The Belmont report: Ethical principles and guidelines for the protection of human subjects of research.* Bethesda, MD; Washington: The Commission; for sale by the Superintendent of Documents, U.S. Government Printing Office.

IRB Initial Review

Although institutions have their own specific IRB forms, the typical initial review form queries:

1. Project title
2. Type of IRB committee requested for review (e.g., behavior and social sciences, biomedical sciences, cancer, and possibly others)
3. Names, titles, degrees, and contact information of principal and coinvestigators, as well as key personnel who will be privy to human subjects information
4. Financial conflict of interest between investigators/institution and funding source
5. Name and contact information for research funding source (e.g., National Institutes of Health [NIH], Centers for Disease Control and Prevention [CDC])
6. Other relevant institutional reviews (e.g., maternal-fetal, radiation, prisoner)
7. Location of research (e.g., domestic, international, multi-site)
8. Summary of research design (usually in fewer than 300 or so words)
9. Scientific background and literature review (justification and importance of the study)
10. Objectives or aims of the research
11. Research methods and activities (usually a checklist including blood draw, publicly available data, observation, stem cell, randomization, surveys, gene transfer, etc.)
12. Required amount of time from each participant
13. Number of participants required (including rationale for the number)
14. Characteristics of the participant population (e.g., ages, decisionally impaired, pregnant women, prisoners, healthy adults, neonates), as well as the rationale for needing this type of population and safeguards for participants who may be vulnerable to coercion or undue influence
15. Participant identification, recruitment, and selection (evidence that the required number of participants is feasible; identification process such as advertising; who will determine eligibility and how it will be determined; explanation of recruitment process and how subjects privacy will be protected; copies of any recruitment materials)
16. Incentives to participate (e.g., type, amount, timing)
17. Alternatives to participation in the research (e.g., available appropriate treatments, therapies, tests, procedures)

18. Informed consent process (e.g., type, procedures, responsible study personnel, minimization of possible coercion, related materials including draft consent forms)

19. Privacy of participants (e.g., provisions to protect, methods to safeguard personally identifiable private information)

20. Confidentiality of data (e.g., type of sensitive information, personnel with access, storage procedures, protection procedures including an NIH Certificate of Confidentiality, plans to keep or destroy at the conclusion of the study)

21. Compliance with the Health Insurance Portability and Accountability Act (HIPAA) research authorization (procedures for handling information subject to the HIPAA privacy rule protecting the confidentiality of subjects' medical information)

22. Reasonably anticipated study benefits to both the participants and society in general

23. Risks, harms, and discomforts (e.g., type, severity, likelihood, and procedures to minimize)

24. Monitoring procedures for data collection that involves more than minimal risk (e.g., responsible personnel, timing, procedures used to evaluate risk, plans for study if risk is greater than anticipated)

25. Assessment of risks and benefits (explanation of why risks are appropriate relative to benefits)

26. Participant costs/reimbursements (monetary costs to participants to participate in research—parking, medication, tests—that will and will not be reimbursed by the study)

27. Application content (initial review form, as well as any number of appendices, including additional information for protecting vulnerable populations, forms, data collection materials, complete grant application, all consent materials, scripts, approval letters, study protocol, etc.)

28. Assurance of principal investigator (PI)/adviser (signature assuring compliance with relevant human subjects protections)

29. Department chair or signatory official (signature indicating that the supervisor of the PI has reviewed the IRB initial review form)

With an emphasis on the regulations for human subject protection, we will discuss the practical applications of the elements of PI qualifications, risk-benefit assessment, and informed consent. We will focus on subject selection and justice in the next section.

Scientific Qualifications

Recall that one directive of the Nuremberg Code is that "the experiment should be conducted only by scientifically qualified personnel." The IRB committee evaluates the scientific qualifications (i.e., relevant degrees and research positions) of investigator(s) and any key personnel. The award of funding and the signature of the investigator's supervisor, in part, confirm the accuracy of this information. Students conducting research must have a qualified adviser who takes the overall responsibility for adhering to human subject guidelines. Protocols submitted by unqualified personnel without the supervision of an adviser would not be approved and permitted to proceed.

Risk-Benefit Assessment

Four relevant criteria for IRB approval are: (1) risks to subjects are reasonable in relation to anticipated benefits; (2) risks to subjects are minimized; (3) when appropriate, there are adequate provisions to protect the privacy of subjects; and (4) when appropriate, the research plan makes adequate provisions for ongoing monitoring for subject safety. These are discussed in the following paragraphs.

Determining if study procedures are ethical or unethical in terms of risks and benefits is rarely straightforward. The results of the assessment are often somewhat ambiguous and are the main focus of the ethics committee. Generally, risks are evaluated and assigned to one of two categories: (1) minimal risk, and (2) greater than minimal risk.

According to the Department of Health and Human Services (2009),

> Minimal risk means that the probability and magnitude of harm or discomfort anticipated in the research are not greater in and of themselves than those ordinarily encountered in daily life or during the performance of routine physical or psychological examinations or tests.

Greater than minimal risks are those that are not ordinarily encountered in daily life or routine exams. Risks greater than minimal require special protections and should be balanced by greater benefits. Harm and discomfort can be physical, psychological, or social in nature. Often, the main challenge of the assessment is determining the likelihood and severity of these.

Examples of risks that would likely be defined as minimal are chest palpitations, blood draws, urine collections, education exams, and psychological tests such as the Minnesota Multiphasic Personality Inventory (MMPI). However, the results of examinations and tests even considered minimal should still be kept private. Examples of risks greater than minimal are spinal taps, experimental medications and procedures, surveys about illegal behaviors, and biopsies. Potential consequences of these research procedures should be adequately anticipated and investigated, and likely effective precautions and safeguards should be instituted.

Minimal precautions are the protection of participants' privacy through confidentiality (never allowing a public link between data and participants' identification) or anonymity (never collecting or recording identifying information). Part of the IRB's assessment procedure is judging the potential effectiveness of safeguards relative to risks. If the safeguards are deemed appropriate, then risks can be said to be "minimized."

Two more general types of potential risk can result from investigators' conflicts of interest with the research and from biased and imprecise research design. Conflicts of interest may exist when investigators have some financial interest in the outcome of their research. They may have a financial ownership in a company testing a drug or device; the company may be funding their research; or study results can be used to develop something within which the investigators' have a financial interest. Conflicts of interest can lead to unnecessary risks to subjects and biased study results. One such risk could result from researchers not disclosing to subjects that effective alternative therapies (outside the scope of the research) are available. Sometimes withholding an effective treatment can be a great risk. A poorly designed study would also put subjects at unnecessary risk because the results of such a study (potential benefits) would likely be useless. Hence, part of the IRB's mandate is to evaluate the potential validity and reliability of the proposed study design.

Two types of benefits are those to the subjects themselves and to society at large. Significant direct benefits would be effective preventions, therapies, and treatments to those undergoing experimental procedures. Clinical trials can and sometimes should (when risks are greater than minimal) achieve direct benefits. Benefits to society at large would be the acquisition of information useful for developing preventions, therapies, and treatments at some point in the future. Such benefits are typically the most that can be expected from nonexperimental designs such as surveys and qualitative methods.

Less obvious benefits are those that do not directly result in health improvements, but may provide subjects with beneficial information, such as diagnoses, test results, and risk evaluations. The provision of resources that help to facilitate health improvement, such as referrals, discounted or free services, and information about treatment options, would be important benefits to subjects. It should be noted that monetary incentives are NOT considered benefits to subjects. Incentives are more appropriately called compensation—payment for the subject's time taken from a job or other productive activity, and reimbursement for travel and other expenses. Incentives should compensate and should not be valued as "awards" at a magnitude that could be coercive. For a prisoner, a pack of cigarettes might even be seen as coercive if they have no other access to the pack.

Voluntary Informed Consent

In the words of the NCPHSBBR (1979),

> An autonomous person is an individual capable of deliberation about personal goals and of acting under the direction of such deliberations. To respect autonomy is to give weight to autonomous persons' considered opinions and choices while refraining from obstructing their actions unless they are clearly detrimental to others.

Unfettered deliberation requires three elements in the consent process: (1) information, (2) comprehension, and (3) voluntariness. These elements should be emphasized in the consent form and process.

A consent form template is presented in **Figure 4–3**. The template provides suggested wording for required concepts that would be generic to any study, and indicates, but leaves blank, required concepts whose details will vary across studies. The consent form should be clearly written and free of ambiguity. The reading and comprehension levels of potential subjects should be considered when drafting the form. Computer programs that determine the reading level of the draft form should be used before finalizing the form.

As shown in the template, information about the study is provided in the purpose (significance and goal) of the study, procedures/tasks (what will be asked of the subject), duration (time commitment of the subject), risks and benefits, and incentives. This is the necessary information for subjects to be "informed" in their decision whether or not to participate.

For subjects to effectively deliberate with the given information, they must clearly understand the information. The probability of comprehension is maximized with clear and appropriate wording about study information. Subjects with limited comprehension and decision-making ability may need the help of a more capable person (outside the study team) who can make a decision on their behalf, with their best interests taking priority. The signature line for authorized consent is shown in Figure 4–3. More specific

IRB Protocol Number:
IRB Application Date:
Version:

[Institution] Consent to Participate in Research

Study Title:

Researcher:

Sponsor:

This is a consent form for research participation. It contains important information about this study and what to expect if you decide to participate.

Your participation is voluntary.

Please consider the information carefully. Feel free to ask questions before making your decision whether or not to participate. If you decide to participate, you will be asked to sign this form and will receive a copy of the form.

Purpose:

Procedures/Tasks:

Duration:

You may leave the study at any time. If you decide to stop participation in the study, there will be no penalty to you, and you will not lose any benefits to which you are otherwise entitled. Your decision will not affect your future relationship with [Institution].

Risks and Benefits:

Confidentiality:

Efforts will be made to keep your study-related information confidential. Outside the study, your name will not be linked to your data. One year after the publication of study results, your identifying information will be destroyed. However, during the conduct of the study, there may be circumstances where your study-related information must be released. For example, personal information regarding your participation in this study may be disclosed if required by state law. Also, your records may be reviewed by the following groups (as applicable to the research):

- Office for Human Research Protection or other federal, state, or international regulatory agencies;
- [Institution] Institutional review board;
- The sponsor or agency (if any) supporting the study.

Incentives:

Participants Rights:

You may refuse to participate in this study without penalty or loss of benefits to which you are otherwise entitled. If you are a student or employee at [Institution], your decision will not affect your grades or employment status.

FIGURE 4–3 (*continued*)

If you choose to participate in the study, you may discontinue participation at any time without penalty or loss of benefits. By signing this form, you do not give up any personal legal rights you may have as a participant in this study.

An institutional review board responsible for human subjects research at [Institution] reviewed this research project and found it to be acceptable, according to applicable state and federal regulations and [Institution] policies designed to protect the rights and welfare of participants in research.

Contacts and Questions:

For questions, concerns, or complaints about the study you may contact _____ (PI).

For questions about your rights as a participant in this study or to discuss other study-related concerns or complaints with someone who is not part of the research team, you may contact _____ in the Office of Responsible Research Practices at 1-800-XXX-XXXX.

If you are injured as a result of participating in this study or for questions about a study-related injury, you may contact _____.

Signing the consent form:

I have read (or someone has read to me) this form and I am aware that I am being asked to participate in a research study. I have had the opportunity to ask questions and have had them answered to my satisfaction. I voluntarily agree to participate in this research.

I am not giving up any legal rights by signing this form. I will be given a copy of this form.

_____
Printed name of subject

_____
Signature of subject

_____ AM/PM
Date and time

_____
**Printed name of person authorized
to consent for subject (if applicable)**

_____
**Signature of authorized person to
consent for subject**

_____ AM/PM
_____
Relationship to subject

Date and time

Investigator/Research Staff

I have explained the research to the participant or his/her representative before requesting the signature(s) above. A copy of this form has been given to the participant or his/her representative.

_____
Printed name of person obtaining consent

_____
Signature of person obtaining consent

_____ AM/PM
Date and time

FIGURE 4–3 Behavioral/Social Science Study Consent Form Template

Source: Modified from the IRB consent form template at the Ohio State University (http://orrp.osu.edu/irb/consent/#consent).

information about this process and when it is appropriate are discussed in the next section.

The consent process should also include an assessment of potential subjects' comprehension of the study goals and procedures. Research staff with the responsibility of obtaining consent should be trained on methods of assessment. One method is to query subjects about various aspects of the study. Ideally, subjects should be asked to state the study purpose and procedures in their own words. Another method is to judge potential participants' comprehension based on the nature of their questions about the study. Questions should be "informed" and not show a basic misunderstanding about the study.

Once the study is fully explained and understood by the participant, he or she should be free to consent or decline. The relevant information about voluntariness is included in the section about participant rights in Figure 4–3. Subjects are told that they can refuse or withdraw from the study without penalty or loss of benefits. Their consent to participate in the study does not then disregard their relevant personal legal right. The IRB should determine that coercion (force) and undue influence (incentives of a magnitude that is difficult to refuse) are absent. If study personnel have any question about whether or not consent is being given voluntarily, they should encourage the potential participant to discuss the study with a third party, one who is not connected with the study and mandated with protection of research subjects. Relevant contact information should be included in the consent form.

It should be noted at this point that legal minors (younger than age 18 years) and adults with diminished capacity to "deliberate about personal goals" cannot give consent on their own behalf. Their agreement to participate is called "assent" and is not enough to enroll them in the study. In these cases, parents or guardians must give consent or permission for minors, and authorized personnel (caregivers, family members) must give consent or permission for those with diminished capacity. More information about these and other special needs is presented in the next section.

SPECIAL NEEDS FOR PROTECTION

In this section, we will discuss the requirement of justice in research. Justice refers to the fair treatment of disadvantaged participants. Most generally, the use of such participants in the study must be justified to the IRB. To the extent possible, competent adults should be used in research with more than minimal risk. There must be compelling scientific and logical reasons to include less advantaged persons. (Recall the Willowbrook study described earlier in this chapter.) If their inclusion is sufficiently justified, less competent subjects should be given additional protections of their rights.

Populations in need of special protection include pregnant women, human fetuses, and neonates; prisoners; and children. The NIH has additional detailed regulations for these populations (DHHS, 2009). Other groups in need of special protection are decisionally impaired adults and non-English-speaking persons. Additional protections address the limited or disadvantaged circumstances of these special populations.

Obviously, human fetuses and neonates cannot consent or assent to research participation. Their protections are overseen by their mother. For such research to be approved, additional conditions must be met and effectively communicated to the mother. For example, preclinical studies of pregnant animals should be conducted first, as appropriate. Researchers cannot intervene or influence in any way the outcome of the pregnancy or the viability of the neonate. The pregnant woman and/or her fetus/neonate should directly benefit from the research.

The issue of voluntary consent is a special circumstance for prisoner populations. Coercion can come from or be perceived to come from prison personnel, and undue influence can be unanticipated. To avoid the perception of coercion, prison personnel are not permitted to be part of the selection process. In addition, eligible prisoners must be chosen for the study randomly. The consent process must also make it clear to prisoners that study participation will not influence any decisions about parole.

In the determination of appropriate incentives, the prisoners' specific living conditions should be considered. Incentives such as quality food and opportunities for earnings in prison may be worth more in a prison setting than they would be outside. Even participation itself as an escape from the boredom of incarceration can be a weighty incentive. Care should be taken to understand the true magnitude of incentives from the prisoners' perspective so as to not exert undue influence to participate.

Risks should not be greater than those that would be accepted by nonprisoner volunteers. Consent language should be understandable to the prison populations. The focus of the research must be specific to "conditions particularly affecting the prisoners as a class" (DHHS, 2009), such as processes of incarceration and health, and other problems experienced by prisoners in excess of those experienced by the general population. IRB committees that review and monitor research on prisoners are required to include a prisoner or prisoner representative.

The use of children in research should be avoided unless scientifically justified and directly relevant to the focus of research. When appropriate, the testing of drugs and medical procedures should first be conducted on adults. Children are "persons who have not attained the legal age for consent to treatment or procedures involved in the research, under the applicable law of the jurisdiction in which the research will be conducted" (DHHS, 2009). Generally, the legal age of consent is 18 years, but exceptions exist depending on the focus of the study relative to appropriate laws. Children can assent or agree to participate, but their legal consent must come in the form of permission from their parents or guardians. When the research involves greater than minimal risk, permission from both parents must be obtained when possible.

In some circumstances, parental consent can be waived for studies. In situations where parental or guardian consent is not likely to be protective (e.g., neglected or abused children), permission can be waived given that an alternative protective mechanism is provided for the child. For example, research on hepatitis C virus (HCV) risk among young injection drug users has been undertaken by Susan Bailey with permission to waive parental consent for minors because many have extremely unhealthy relationships with their parents or guardians. In lieu of parental consent, potential subjects were given contact information for a service organization that provides support for troubled and homeless youth. They were encouraged to call the organization if they have any questions or concerns about study participation. It is important that the protective mechanism is independent of the research team, institution, and funder, and has no conflict of interest with the study.

Decisionally impaired adults and non-English-speaking persons also require special protections. The former group should only be included in research if the focus of the study is specific to the situation of the group (e.g., effective therapies for adults with traumatic head injuries, drug treatments for schizophrenia). When possible, similar studies should first be conducted with animals and competent adults. When decisionally impaired groups are used in research, persons with proper authorization for their consent must provide such consent. Authorized persons would be those with professional experience with the particular disability of the potential subjects. They should have no conflicts of interest with the study.

Foreign or domestic studies of non-English-speaking persons must develop all consent and other study materials in the appropriate native language(s). Care must be taken to develop a true translation of materials from English, when researchers are English speaking. Ideally, bilingual experts in the appropriate language, say Spanish, would translate the English version of materials developed by investigators. Then another bilingual expert would translate the Spanish version back to English to assure their comparability. In addition to language issues, culturally relevant norms and traditions must be respected and reflected in all study procedures.

More often than not, unanticipated problems arise in the course of a research study. For this reason, the IRB provides periodic (typically yearly) review of study progress and outcomes, and may require protocol changes or even study termination in the event of unforeseen risks or other negative outcomes. Part of this monitoring process involves strict and honest record keeping by both the study team and the IRB. Human subject materials are also reported to funding agencies or other relevant government agencies. These layers of oversight require a great deal of time and effort from study personnel, but the protection of human subjects in light of their treatment historically certainly justifies the effort.

CONCLUSION

The boundary between what is ethical and unethical in research is often blurred. Not only are consequences and outcomes sometimes unanticipated, but there is often, if not always a subjective component to the evaluation of risks and benefits. For example, the distinction between minimal and greater than minimal risk is not always clear and universally agreed upon. Efforts to minimize risk may not always be successful. Direct benefits may not always be achieved at the magnitude expected or even at all. These are the reasons for careful study design in accordance with human subjects regulations and ongoing multilayered reviews.

Aside from the extreme cases of risk and benefit, there is no universal definition of ethical research. However, the following practices, sometimes depending on the focus and procedures of the study, push or cross the ethical boundaries (Kimmel, 1979). It is prudent to avoid these in research designs.

1. Involving people without their knowledge or consent
2. Coercing people to participate

3. Withholding information about the true nature of the research
4. Deceiving the participant
5. Inducing participants to commit acts that diminish their self-esteem
6. Violating rights of self-determination
7. Exposing individuals to physical or emotional stress
8. Invading privacy
9. Withholding benefits
10. Not treating participants with respect

The old adage to treat others as you would want to be treated is probably the most reliable compass to follow in conducting ethical research. Given a certain probable benefit, would you be willing to be exposed to the potential risks? What if you were consenting for your grandparents, siblings, children, spouse, and so on?

VOCABULARY

Assent	Institutional review	Parental consent
Autonomy	board (IRB)	Risk-benefit assessment
Belmont Report	Justice	Tuskegee syphilis study
Beneficence	Minimal risk	Voluntary consent
Coercion	Minor	Willowbrook hepatitis
Deception	National Research Act	study
Decisionally impaired	Nuremberg Code	
Declaration of Helsinki	NY Jewish Chronic	
Incentives	Disease	
Informed consent	Hospital study	

STUDY QUESTIONS AND EXERCISES

1. Access the National Institutes of Health (NIH) website (www.nih.gov) and complete the human subjects protection certification program. Print the certificate with your name on it.
2. Describe the backgrounds and expertise of the members of your institution's IRB.
3. Describe a hypothetical study that would not be approved by an IRB. What specific protections are violated in the study?

4. Summarize a famous study (e.g., prison study, shock study) that pushed or crossed the ethical boundary of human subjects' protection. What specific protections were compromised or violated in the study?

5. Fill out the IRB application for your institution's study review. Use either your particular study design or imagine a hypothetical study. (See your institution's IRB webpage for forms and instructions.)

6. Draft an informed consent form for your real or hypothetical study. Be sure to include all the important elements, and check the reading level to maximize subjects' comprehension. If your design requires consent forms from individuals other than subjects (e.g., parents/guardians, caregivers, institutional representatives), draft these as well. Indicate the purpose of each form.

REFERENCES

Curran, W. J. (1973). The Tuskegee syphilis study. *The New England Journal of Medicine, 289*(14), 730–731.

Department of Health and Human Services. (2009). *Code of Federal Regulations Title 45 Public Welfare, Part 46 Protection of Human Subjects,* revision effective July 14, 2009.

Katz, J., Capron, A. M., & Glass, E. S. (1972). *Experimentation with human beings: The authority of the investigator, subject, professions, and state in the human experimentation process.* New York: Russell Sage Foundation.

Kimmel, A. J. (1979). Ethics and human subjects research: A delicate balance. *The American Psychologist, 34*(7), 633–635.

Krugman, S. (1986). The Willowbrook hepatitis studies revisited: Ethical aspects. *Reviews of Infectious Diseases, 8*(1), 157–162.

Lind, J. (1757). *A treatise on the scurvy* (2nd ed.). London: A. Millar.

National Commission for the Protection of Human Subjects of Biomedical and Behavioral Research. (1979). *The Belmont report: Ethical principles and guidelines for the protection of human subjects of research.* Bethesda, MD; Washington, DC: Government Printing Office

World Medical Association. (1964). *Declaration of Helsinki—ethical principles for medical research involving human subjects.* Helsinki, Finland: 18th WMA General Assembly.

CHAPTER 5

Formulating a Research Question

LEARNING OBJECTIVES

By the end of this chapter the reader will be able to:

- Distinguish between types of research questions based on different study designs.
- Generate ideas for research questions.
- Formulate an operationalizable research question.

CHAPTER OUTLINE

Research requires a question for which no ready answer is available.
—Unknown

INTRODUCTION

A research question is the organizing principle for an entire study. It clarifies exactly what the researcher wants to describe or explain. It bridges the gap between a research problem and a detailed plan for study design and analysis. The methodological approach and study design stem directly from the focus of the research question, which is a specific component of the research problem. The operationalization of the research problem can be expressed as research questions, objectives, or hypotheses. The choice of question, objective, or hypothesis depends, in large part, on what is known about the research problem. Objectives and research questions are the best choice in situations where little information and relevant research are available and where the main purpose of the study is to identify or describe characteristics or examine relationships. Hypotheses are the best choice if the researcher is testing a component of a theory or examining a causal relationship. Typically, answers to researcher questions generate hypotheses to be tested.

TYPES OF RESEARCH QUESTIONS

There are three basic types of research questions: (1) descriptive, (2) association, and (3) causal. Descriptive questions are largely observational, with a focus on the "who, where, and when" of the health phenomenon. Association or correlation questions examine risk factors for the health problem. Causal questions demonstrate the determinants of health phenomena and test the efficacy of deterrents in the form of preventions and interventions. **Figure 5–1** demonstrates the three basic types of research questions.

Descriptive

Descriptive questions can be addressed in case studies, case series, cross-sectional, case-control, and cohort studies. The main objective is to describe the extent of the health phenomena, who experiences it, and where and when it occurs. For example, consider questions about the body mass index (BMI) of Americans. Descriptive questions aim to describe the trend of BMI. Questions usually begin with "How often," "How much," "What number," or "What percentage." For example:

> "How many Americans are overweight?"
> "What percentage of Americans have a high BMI?"
> "How many American men and women are overweight?"

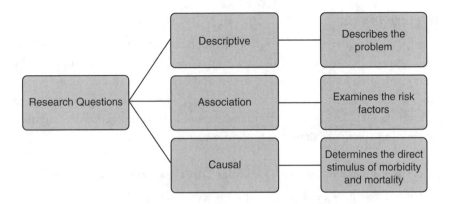

FIGURE 5–1 Types of Research Questions

Again, the focus of the question must be specific enough to operationalize or translate into a measurable process. Concepts like "overweight" and "high BMI" must be defined specifically so they can be observed in a consistent and true manner.

Example: Incidence and Prevalence of Childhood Type 2 Diabetes

Type 2 diabetes in children is a "newly recognized" pediatric disease. Historically, diabetes mellitus in children and adolescents was believed to be primarily Type 1. However, cases of youth Type 2 diabetes have been noted since 1979, but the prevalence was too low to stimulate closer examination. There are currently no nationwide epidemiological data focusing on Type 2 diabetes in children. However, clinic-based reports and regional studies consistently emphasize the increasing prevalence of this emerging health problem. For example, in Cincinnati, Ohio, medical charts of diagnosed diabetes cases from 1982 to 1995 were reviewed, and the incidence of Type 2 diabetes in 10- to 19-year-old subjects increased from 0.7/100,000 in 1982 to 7.2/100,000 in 1994 (Pinhas-Hamiel, Dolan, Daniels, et al., 1996). These results are intended to characterize the problem and generate causal hypotheses to be tested in more sophisticated study designs.

Historically, adult Pima Indians in Arizona are known to have a high prevalence of Type 2 diabetes. Researchers looked at Pima Indian youth (from 1992 to 1996) in Arizona and calculated a prevalence of Type 2 diabetes of 22.3 per 1,000 population 10 to 14 years old and 50.9 per 1,000 in the 15- to 19-year age group (Dabelea, Hanson, Bennett, et al., 1998). These results focused on person characteristics in describing Type 2 diabetes.

Determinants

Determinants are essentially causes of health phenomena: bacteria, viruses, chemicals, stress, carcinogens, alcohol abuse, and so on. Determinants are suggested by results focusing on associations in cohort and case-control studies. Their precise role as causes is tested in experimental studies. These types of questions try to answer the "why" and "how" of a phenomenon. For example, consider questions examining potential risk factors for cardiovascular diseases.

Example: Obesity and Cardiovascular Disease (CVD) Risk Factors

Obesity levels have been associated with several adverse health outcomes. It is widely known that obesity can impact work capacity and fitness level of individuals. A prospective cohort study of firefighters was conducted to examine the associations between obesity and other cardiovascular disease risk factors (Soteriades, Hauser, Kawachi, et al., 2005). Results of this study showed that the rates of obesity increased over time, and obese firefighters were more likely to have hypertension, and low high-density lipoprotein (HDL) cholesterol. Also, firefighters with extreme obesity had an average of 2.1 CVD risk factors compared to 1.5 for normal weight firefighters. These results support an association between obesity and CVD risk factors.

A case-control study of colorectal cancer evaluated the association between BMI and risk of colorectal cancer (Campbell, Jacobs, Ulrich, et al., 2010). Subjects with this type of cancer were matched with unaffected sex-matched siblings to evaluate these associations. The results of this study indicated a significant positive association between BMI and risk of colorectal cancer (odds ratio [OR] = 1.24, 95% confidence interval [CI] = 1.15 to 1.34). Lower risk estimates were reported for women compared to males (OR = 1.34 vs. OR = 1.79).

Deterrents

The ultimate goal of epidemiological research is to prevent or control morbidity and mortality. It is important to describe the distribution of a problem and identify the risk factors associated with it. However, knowing the true cause of the problem facilitates the implementation of strategies to prevent or reduce health problems. Causal questions aim to determine the direct stimulants (exposures or independent variables) of morbidity and mortality (outcomes or dependent variables). These questions can be addressed and the efficacy of deterrents evaluated in clinical or community trials.

Example: Diabetes Prevention Trial: Effect of Lifestyle Changes on Prevention of Type 2 Diabetes

Research has established that the prevalence of Type 2 diabetes is increasing and that behavioral and environmental risk factors play a significant role. The diabetes prevention program in this evaluation study tested the efficacy of modest weight loss through dietary changes and increases in physical activity to prevent or delay the onset of Type 2 diabetes (Tuomilehto, Lindström, Eriksson, et al., 2001). A clinical trial was designed. Subjects in the treatment group received intensive dietary advice (lower total fat intake, increased fiber intake) and physical activity motivations (30 minutes/day). The control group was given general oral and written information about diet and exercise at baseline and at each annual visit. The follow-up lasted 3.2 years, and results at the end point indicated that the risk of diabetes was 58% lower in the intervention group than the control group (95% CI, 48%–66%, $p < 0.001$). These results also demonstrate that Type 2 diabetes is the direct result of suboptimal lifestyle factors.

GENERATING RESEARCH QUESTIONS

How are research questions generated? They emerge through the refinement of research problems or ideas. Potential sources of research questions include observations in everyday life, findings from relevant studies, practical issues in the field of study, and theory (Clark & Creswell, 2010). These four methods for generating researchable questions occur in the initial stages of the research process. Each is explained in detail in the sections that follow.

Everyday Life

One of the best ways to generate research questions is through observations and experiences in professional life. For example, dietitians may note that some people are successful in losing weight while others are not. Some people diet but are very sedentary, while others diet as well as incorporate physical activity into their lifestyle. Observations such as these, although essentially anecdotal, suggest research questions. Based on these example observations, researchers could ask if a low-carbohydrate diet is associated with weight loss, if water consumption is associated with losing weight, or if there is a relationship between physical activity duration and weight loss.

Practical Issues in the Field

Every profession has certain chronic issues that require answers to multiple complex research questions. For example, the public health sector is currently faced with the epidemic of global obesity. There is a keen interest in effective strategies to prevent the incidence and reduce the prevalence of obesity. Case study observations may suggest that certain lower socioeconomic groups are at a higher risk for obesity and related consequences compared to higher social classes. These observations can stimulate cohort and case-control studies and evaluation of strategies to cause an equal distribution of healthy and affordable food supply. An example of a relevant research question is: "Is food insecurity more prevalent among African Americans compared to Caucasians?"

Relevant Studies

The review and synthesis of findings from previous studies is a good source of research ideas to generate research questions. Reviewing the literature of studies helps to identify the gaps in knowledge. These gaps can be addressed in research questions for future studies. Often reviewing and critiquing research articles helps identify the limitations of a particular study, and these limitations can open a door for generating research questions. Most simply, research questions can replicate, expand, or strengthen the results of previous studies. New studies can address conflicting results in two or more previous studies. New research questions can also test the external validity of published research (e.g., Do successful nutrition education lesson plans for Caucasian populations also work for Latino populations?).

Theory

Epidemiologic theory is the collection of related integrated principles or laws that describe, explain, predict, or control health phenomena. Theory helps generate hypotheses. Theory integrates current knowledge to develop causal principles, and research tests and modifies or expands these principles. For example, Albert Bandura (1986) introduced the concept of self-efficacy in the context of behavior modification. In other words, behavior change is facilitated by a personal sense of control. If an individual has high self-efficacy (confidence) that he or she can take action to solve a problem, then that person will likely be successful in that behavior. Research studies have tested and found support for this theory in the context of changes in health-related diet and exercise behaviors.

Theories are an excellent starting point for developing research questions as they provide a set of interrelated concepts, definitions, and relations among variables in order to explain and/or predict the situations. Two key terms used in theories are *concepts* and *constructs*; concepts are the main elements and constructs operationalize the key concepts (Glanz & Bishop, 2010; Glanz, Lewis, & Rimer, 1996; Glanz, Rimer, & Lewis, 2002). Application of theory allows a researcher to conduct systematic assessment of the problem, its causes, and possible solutions. Theories can be used during various stages of planning, implementing, or even evaluating research interventions. Theories help answer the "Why, What, and How" questions. In other words, theory can help answer questions such as why some people do not make healthy food choices or what one needs to know before developing an intervention program, and it can help understand how to design successful public health programs or interventions (Glanz & Bishop, 2010; Glanz, Lewis, & Rimer, 1996; Glanz, Rimer, & Lewis, 2002).

Theories help explain behavior and suggest ways to achieve behavior change. An explanatory theory like a health belief model helps describe and identify why a problem exists. These theories help predict behaviors and help search for modifiable factors like knowledge, attitudes, self-efficacy, social support, and lack of resources. A change theory, or theories of action, help the development of interventions. These theories can also form the basis for evaluation (Glanz & Bishop, 2010).

The four most commonly used theoretical models of health behavior are:

1. *Health belief model*—people's beliefs about risk for a certain disease or health problem and their perception of benefits of taking action to prevent it influences their readiness to take action.
2. *Transtheoretical model or stages of change*—this theory proposes that people are at different stages of readiness to adopt healthful behaviors.
3. *Social cognitive theory*—emphasizes that people not only learn through their own experiences, but also via observational learning, reinforcement, self-control, and self-efficacy.
4. *Social ecological model*—helps understand factors affecting behavior and guides the development of intervention programs through social environments. Theories can help generate descriptive, determinant, and deterrent questions.

Example: Examining the Etiology of Childhood Obesity: The IDEA Study

The increasing prevalence of childhood obesity is a major public health concern. Research indicates that childhood obesity tracks into adulthood and results in increased risk for cardiovascular diseases, diabetes, and hypertension. In addition, the economic costs associated with obesity are also increasing. A study by Youfa Wang and colleagues indicated that obesity will account for more than 16% of all healthcare expenditures by 2030 (Wang, Beydoun, Liang, et al., 2008). Causes of childhood obesity are complex and multifaceted; hence, prevention strategies need to focus on multiple levels. A socioecological framework that focuses on multiple levels of influence, potential predictors of development of obesity in youth, mutable factors that can be examined in future community-level health promotion interventions, and predictive factors and their relationship with body mass index was developed to be tested in this longitudinal study. Leslie Lytle's (2009) research paper proposed a conceptual model for etiology of childhood obesity.

Lytle's proposed model provides an opportunity to test many research questions. Researchers can test the correlates and predictors of weight status and the potential interactive effects of the factors assessed at each level of the conceptual model and can evaluate the mediating and moderating effects of the contextual, behavioral, and biological factors. Modifiers like family status and school or neighborhood situation may also be studied as potential effect modifiers.

Secondary Databases or Secondary Data Analysis

Secondary analysis of publically available health data is an efficient and cost-effective mechanism for generating a research project. Developing research questions for secondary data analysis can be achieved in two ways: (1) finding research questions to fit an existing data set, or (2) finding an existing data set to fit the specific research questions.

It is very likely that researchers will begin with a research question and then search for the perfect data set that will allow analysis of that question. Once the question is formulated, the researcher should conduct a thorough literature review to determine the predictor and outcome variables that will help answer the research question or might influence the research question. After an analysis of the literature, the next step is to locate the potential databases that will help answer the research question. The question might need to be refined in terms of the data available. Another option for researchers is to start by selecting a publically available secondary data set, and then formulate a research question based on the variables present in the data set (Bibb, 2007; Boslaugh, 2007).[*]

Example: National Health and Nutrition Examination Survey (NHANES)

If as a researcher you decide to work with NHANES data set, it is important that you make yourself familiar with the data set. You will need to ask questions such as:

What type of data is collected by NHANES?

What was the process of data collection (in-person interviews, telephone interviews, etc.)?

---

[*]Sara Boslaugh's *Secondary data sources for public health: A practical guide* (2007) is an excellent reference for information on secondary databases.

What questions are asked during this survey?

How are the responses coded?

When was the data collected?

What age groups are included in this data set?

and many more. You must understand what cleaning or recoding procedures have been applied to the data. The NHANES website provides detailed information on the process of data collection and maintenance of data (http://www.cdc.gov/nchs/nhanes/nhanes_questionnaires.htm). Once you feel comfortable with the data set, you can start refining your research ideas or generating research questions. For example, you are interested in studying childhood obesity and related information. One of the most straightforward research questions that comes to mind is: "What is the prevalence of childhood obesity among 6 to 11 year olds?" You are also interested in comparing the prevalence of childhood obesity across the years (use NHANES data sets from across the years): Does the prevalence of childhood obesity differ by gender and race? Is there a link between socioeconomic status and childhood obesity?

An interesting article by Huffman, Kanikireddy, and Patel (2010) used NHANES III data set to evaluate the association between parental study and childhood overweight. NHANES III was an appropriate data set for this study, as it facilitated matching children's data with their parents' data. The authors extracted data from NHANES III data set, matching parents with children using their family sequence numbers in the adult and youth data files. A new data set focusing on matched parents with children was formed. Two hundred and nineteen (219) households with single parents and 780 dual-parent households were analyzed for variables of interest. Findings indicated that children from single-parent households were significantly more overweight ($p < 0.01$) and had higher total caloric and saturated fat intake ($p < 0.05$).

FORMULATING THE SPECIFIC RESEARCH QUESTION

Research questions often begin with the review of previous relevant studies. Researchers narrow the scope of research questions by clearly defining the goal for a study, consulting colleagues, and linking a question to specific hypotheses or working concepts of research. A few things to consider in writing good research questions follow.

Components of a Good Research Question

Components of a good research question should include "who" (subjects or units being assessed), "what" (the exposure and outcome of interest), and "how" (correlation or causal relationship). In other words, the well developed research question will identify the group or population of subjects, study parameters (cause, correlates, intervention, etc.), outcomes of interest, and the types of relationships examined. Researchers identify the key characteristics of participants, study site, major variables (independent, dependent, and control), and questions. Some examples of strong research questions are: "What is the association between severe malnutrition and mortality?" and "What is the incidence of depression in elderly subjects at a long-term care facility?"

A good research question should be ethical, clear, feasible, and significant. To be ethical, the risk/harm (physical or emotional) to the subjects or population should be outweighed by the benefit of the study to them and the field. To be clear, key terms in the research study should be specifically defined in a manner that can be observable and measurable. The level of detail should be specific enough that the elements can be replicated by others. To be feasible, the proposed research question should be operationalizable, and important and appropriate components should be available. Components of feasibility include adequate money, time, manpower, and resources (e.g., access to subjects, accurate measures). As far as significance, answers to the proposed research question should make a meaningful contribution to the field, the human condition, or practice of patient care. Potential causes should be supported or refuted, and interventions should be demonstrated as effective or not.

One commonly used acronym to define the characteristics of good research questions is FINER, where **F** stands for feasible, **I** for interesting, **N** for novel, **E** for ethical, and **R** for relevant (Farrugia, Petrisor, Farrokhyar, et al., 2010). Distinguishing levels of inquiry is a popular technique used to write good research questions. At level 1, the factor of interest is isolated. At level 2, relationships between factors are examined. At level 3, causal relationships are inferred or tested.

Level 1—Factor-Isolating Questions

This level is used when little information is available on the topic of interest. The "what" questions are answered often by analyzing one health factor. Exploratory or descriptive study designs are best for this level of inquiry. For example, "What is the incidence of Type 2 diabetes in children and adolescents in the United States?"

Level 2—Factor-Relating Questions

Level 2 inquiry is used to explore the relationships between two or more variables. These can be descriptive characteristics (e.g., sociodemographic characteristics) or risk factors (e.g., stress). Cohort and case-control studies are appropriate for this level of inquiry. For example, "What is the association between total fat intake (in grams) and weight gain?"

Level 3—Situation-Producing Questions

Level 3 inquiry is used to test causal relationships between two or more variables. More specifically, this highest level is used to predict or anticipate an outcome (dependent variable) due to causal factors (independent variables). Level 3 inquiry is mainly used in experimental studies that test hypotheses. Hypotheses can be written in an associative (correlation), null (no relationship), or directional (positive or negative) format. For example, "There is no difference in the prevalence of obesity between 10- to 16-year-old African American and Caucasian boys."

CONCLUSION

This chapter introduces the three different types of research questions. These questions stem from the research problem and direct the research design and plan for data collection and analysis. Research questions can focus on incidence or prevalence (descriptive questions), associations or risk factors (associative questions), and determinants and deterrents (causal questions). The selection of study design is based completely on the type of research question. For example, a cross-sectional study is well suited to study the incidence of obesity in children. In designing research questions, it is essential to clarify the target population, exposure, and outcome of interest, and how the concepts are assessed. A clear and concise research question is essential to a successful study.

VOCABULARY

Conceptual model	Deterrents	Secondary data analysis
Descriptive questions	FINER	Theory
Determinants	Research question	

STUDY QUESTIONS AND EXERCISES

1. Describe how the research question bridges the gap between the research problem and the study design. Give specific novel examples in your description.

2. Give specific and novel examples of the three basic types of research questions.

3. Describe the four methods for generating research questions. Give specific and novel examples in your description.

4. Describe the elements of a good research question.

5. What types of questions usually begin with "How much," or "What percentage"?
   a. Descriptive
   b. Association
   c. Causal

6. A study asks, "What is the frequency of fast food consumption in urban black adolescents?" What kind of research question is this?
   a. Descriptive
   b. Association
   c. Causal

7. One of the major problems our nation currently is faced with is increasing rates of childhood obesity. Below is a very generic scenario of this problem.

   Scenario:

   Childhood obesity rates are increasing in the United States and around the world. Lifestyle behaviors (diet, exercise, sedentary behavior) are considered to be significant contributors to this problem.

   Based on this problem statement, address the following:
   a. Design a "descriptive" research question and describe the appropriate study design to answer this question.
   b. Design an "association" research question and describe the appropriate study design.
   c. Design a "causal" research question and describe the appropriate study design.

FURTHER READING

Friis, R. H., & Sellers, T. A. (2009). *Epidemiology for public health practice* (4th ed.). Sudbury, MA: Jones & Bartlett Learning.

REFERENCES

Bandura, A. (1986). *Social foundations of thought and action: A social cognitive theory.* Englewood Cliffs, NJ: Prentice-Hall.

Bibb, S. C. G. (2007). Issues associated with secondary analysis of population health data. *Applied Nursing Research, 20*, 94–99.

Boslaugh, S. (2007). *Secondary data sources for public health: A practical guide.* New York: Cambridge University Press.

Campbell, P. T., Jacobs, E. T., Ulrich, C. M., Figueiredo, J. C., Poynter, J. N., McLaughlin, J. R., et al. (2010). Case–control study of overweight, obesity, and colorectal cancer risk, overall and by tumor microsatellite instability status. *Journal of the National Cancer Institute, 102*, 391–400.

Clark, V. L. P., & Creswell, J. W. (2010). *Understanding research: A consumer's guide.* Upper Saddle River, NJ: Pearson Education.

Dabelea, D., Hanson, R. L., Bennett, P. H., Roumain, J., Knowler, W. C., & Pettitt, D. J. (1998). Increasing prevalence of type II diabetes in American Indian children. *Diabetologia, 41*, 904– 910.

Farrugia, P., Petrisor, B. A., Farrokhyar, F., & Bhandari, M. (2010). Research questions, hypothesis and objectives. *Canadian Journal of Surgery,. 53*(4), 278–281.

Glanz, K., & Bishop, D. B. (2010). The role of behavioral science theory in development and implementation of public health interventions. *Annual Review of Public Health, 31*, 399–418.

Glanz, K., Lewis, F. M., & Rimer, B. K. (Eds.). (1996). *Health behavior and health education: Theory, research, and practice* (2nd ed.). San Francisco: Jossey-Bass.

Glanz, K., Rimer, B. K., & Lewis, F. M. (2002). *Health behavior and health education: Theory, research, and practice* (3rd ed.). San Francisco: Jossey-Bass.

Huffman, F. G., Kanikireddy, S., & Patel, M. (2010). Parenthood—a contributing factor to childhood obesity. *International Journal of Environmental Research and Public Health, 7*, 2800–2810.

Lytle, L. A. (2009). Examining the etiology of childhood obesity: The IDEA study. *American Journal of Community Psychology, 44*(3–4), 338.

Pinhas-Hamiel, O., Dolan, L. M., Daniels, S. R., Standiford, D., Khoury, P. R., Zeitler, P. (1996). Increased incidence of non-insulin-dependent diabetes mellitus among adolescents. *Journal of Pediatrics,128*(5), 608–615.

Soteriades, E. S., Hauser, R., Kawachi, I., Liarokapis, D., Christiani, D. C., & Kales, S. N. (2005). Obesity and cardiovascular disease risk factors in firefighters: A prospective cohort study. *Obesity Research, 13*(10), 1756–1763.

Tuomilehto, J., Lindström, J., Eriksson, J. G., Valle, T. T., Hämäläinen, H., & Ilanne-Parikka, P. (2001). Prevention of type 2 diabetes mellitus by changes in lifestyle among subjects with impaired glucose tolerance. *New England Journal of Medicine, 344*(18),1343–1350.

Wang, Y., Bedoun, M. A., Liang, L., Caballero, B., & Kumanyika, S. K. (2008). Will all Americans become overweight or obese? Estimating the progression and cost of the U.S. obesity epidemic. *Obesity, 16*(10), 2323–2330.

CHAPTER 6

Reviewing the Literature

LEARNING OBJECTIVES

By the end of this chapter the reader will be able to:
- Explain the purposes of the literature review.
- Describe the elements of the review.
- Conduct a literature search.
- Write a literature review.

CHAPTER OUTLINE

Review, Organize, Summarize . . . is that what Review of Literature is?

INTRODUCTION

The literature review is an essential step in the process of conducting research. It is often via the process of reviewing studies (or the "literature") related to the "proposed research" that the research question is formulated, revised, and finalized. The review involves locating and selecting relevant studies, and organizing and summarizing their relevant content. Note the repeated use of the word *relevant*. If the body of prior relevant research is broad, a selective choice of studies should focus on particular target populations, research questions, measures, and so on that are similar to the new study. If the body of research is limited because the new study is one of the first of its kind, then most or all relevant studies can be reviewed. So a broad body of studies warrants a focused review, and a limited body means a general review.

The literature review itself is a summarized document that describes and critiques the past and present state of information about a certain topic. It provides a link between the existing knowledge and the problem of interest. The review organizes the results of prior studies into subtopics according to the themes, such as target populations, study designs, historical period, and so on. In addition to educating the researcher about what is known and not known about the topic of interest, a review of previous studies indicates how others have designed their studies—what research methods have been used and which are a perfect fit for the new study. **Figure 6–1** presents a flow of steps involved in the process of literature review.

A thorough review includes information from books, journal articles, conference papers, government documents, and so on. Regardless of the source of the information, the review facilitates the definition, refinement, and design of the current study. A summary of the strengths and limitations of prior studies guides the researcher in identifying appropriate methodologies as well as their limitations, summarizing contradictory findings, and developing a focused and important hypothesis.

CONDUCTING THE LITERATURE SEARCH

The thorough review includes studies published (and sometimes unpublished) in a variety of sources. The point is to identify all or most of the relevant studies, both well and little known, to focus the research question to address the unknown or uncertain aspects of the research topic.

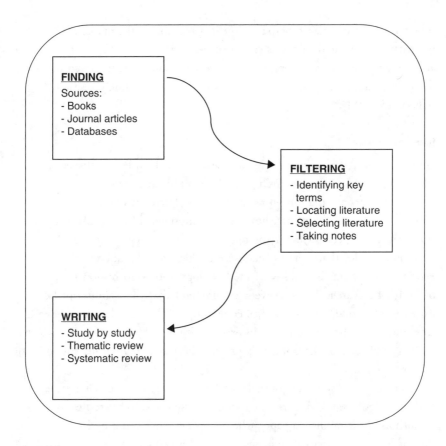

FIGURE 6-1 Flow of Steps Involved in the Process of Literature Review

Sources of Information

Books

Textbooks are great resources for basic theories and concepts that help build a research foundation. Information about methods, measurements, pathophysiology of medical conditions, and statistical tests can be obtained from textbooks. Books can also provide a list of references as a starting point for a branching bibliography where one source cites a source to inspect, which cites another source to inspect, and so on. Books can be obtained from academic libraries. Online catalogs provide a listing of all textbooks available on a particular topic.

Books are a handy source of information, but they are limited in terms of their timeliness. Publishing a book takes approximately 3 to 5 years from the time the author starts writing to the time it is available in the market. Hence, the information presented in books can be as many as 7 years old. In an emerging and evolving field, it is imperative to also review more current and cutting-edge research. Articles in professional journals provide more timely research results (Chatburn, 2011).

Journal Articles

Generally, journal articles are original research-based studies published in peer-reviewed journals. These research journals are published at regular intervals and present current information on research topics. There are a number of journals available across all disciplines; however, the most reliable journals in terms of study rigor are peer-reviewed (or refereed) journals. A peer-reviewed journal publishes articles that start as manuscripts that are subsequently reviewed by experts in the field for quality of methodology and contribution to literature or body of research. The reviewers' recommend that the manuscript be published as submitted, revised, or rejected. Most published articles have undergone substantial revisions in response to expert critiques. This process ensures that articles published in these journals present the result of rigorous studies with minimal biases.

There are two types of journal articles: (1) original research articles, and (2) review articles. Original research articles present results of studies conducted by authors of the published paper, whereas review articles summarize the existing knowledge on a particular topic based on extensive literature searches. Another term used for original research articles is *primary source*, and for review articles is *secondary source*. In the initial stages of a literature review, it is sometimes helpful to use secondary sources (review articles) because they (1) often present an overview of a topic, citing important primary sources; (2) save time—authors have already researched the topic; and (3) provide a list of references that will help in branching bibliographies. However, it should be noted that reviews include thoughts and summarizations made by the author. The summaries represent a particular point of view and may exclude sources that are irrelevant to the author's point of view but are important for the current study. Hence, thoroughly reviewing primary sources in addition to secondary sources is essential (McMillan, 2008).

Databases

Databases are an organized collection of research results. In this era of computers, it is now feasible to have huge databases that store millions and millions of information sources (research studies, articles, etc.). These stored sources provide an efficient and broad-based mechanism for locating information and displaying it in customized formats. The key component of a database is the index, or the method of locating data or information. The most popular medical database categories or formats are bibliographic, citation, and synthesized.

Bibliographic databases are the most commonly used databases, and PubMed is the most popular bibliographic database. This type of database contains information on books, reports, citations, abstracts, and either full-text articles or links to the full-text. PubMed provides the complete citation of the articles, abstracts of articles, and links to full-text articles. Searches can be conducted by author name, article title, journal, year, or keywords that represent the general topic of the studies. Users can save and email their search results.

Citation databases facilitate the tracking of all published research that has been done to date on a particular research topic. Searches are done by study title and authors of the study. ISI Web of Knowledge is one of the most popular citation databases. Synthesized databases are prefiltered records for particular research topics. They provide one of the quickest searches to find the best results relevant to particular research topics. This type of database can be used to identify sources to search in citation databases. However, access to synthesized databases is mostly via subscription and is relatively expensive. Cochrane Collaboration is the leading database in this category. Cochrane Reviews are exhaustive reviews of literature on a given topic. Such reviews can be used as a starting point to locate relevant primary sources of research. Some other examples of synthesized databases are National Guideline Clearinghouse and UpToDate (Chatburn, 2011; Johnson & Christensen, 2008).

Filtering Literature

Just finding literature is not enough. Results of searches should be further limited to what is directly relevant. Searches often produce a lot of articles generally relevant to the area of interest, but inclusion and exclusion criteria should be used to focus the results. The important steps in filtering research are to (1) identify key terms, using correct search strategies, (2) select relevant and good quality research, and (3) take notes on the key aspects of each article (Clark & Creswell, 2010).

Identifying Key Terms or Keywords

As a way to direct the initial and subsequent searches, keywords are entered in the actual search program. These can be words or short phrases. The more accurate the keywords, the more focused and relevant are the search results. In fact, authors of journal articles are asked to provide the publisher with keywords that they believe best characterize the important features of their articles. Helpful key terms indicate the target population of the study (e.g., youth, hospital patients, immigrants), the overall study methodology (e.g., case-control, randomized controlled trial, ethnography), the exposure or risk factor of interest (e.g., obesity, low-socioeconomic status, living near a nuclear power plant), the outcome of interest (e.g., diabetes, alcohol abuse, pancreatic cancer), measures (e.g., BMI, stress, zip codes), and analytic strategy (e.g., life table, logistic regression, content analysis). Some or all of these types of keywords may be appropriate, but the exposure and outcome are probably indispensible.

The best strategy for choosing keywords is to think about these aspects of the study at hand (target population, exposure, etc.) and make lists of representative terms. Then search on the best of these. As the search progresses, more or perhaps all of these terms can be used until the desired number of relevant studies are identified.

Locating Literature

Locating literature online is not a difficult job; however, using efficient and effective strategies for searching literature is essential. It is important to use academic libraries and electronic databases, which include primarily peer-reviewed work. Academic libraries are great resources for searching reliable published literature and offer a large collection of materials, physically, as well as online catalogs of their holdings. Another great way to locate resources is through electronic databases. Some of the most common databases for health and behavioral research are ERIC (Education Resources Information Center), PubMed, EBSCO, and Google Scholar.

Selecting Literature

Most literature searches produce a large body of reference material. At this point, it is necessary to scan the literature and determine if individual studies are relevant for the research topic at hand. A quick scan of each article in terms of title, abstract, and major headings in the study helps determine if the source is relevant for use. The initial scan can be accomplished within the search database. Even when full-text articles are not available through the database, abstracts of relatively recent articles typically are. Information provided in the abstract is often enough to determine if the study is likely relevant and worthy of viewing the full article. For these, full-text articles should be retrieved and read thoroughly for information to include in the note-taking process.

Taking Notes

Once all relevant full-text articles are collected, the next step is to review, organize, and summarize these articles. Organizing and summarizing articles makes it easy to use and locate the information when writing the literature review. The exclusion of irrelevant studies is another important outcome of note taking. There are several methods for organizing and summarizing results of study reviews. Summaries in tabular formats are often easy to prepare and efficient to use.

Table 6–1 presents an in-progress example of a tabular format for organizing and summarizing research results. The first column is the "study" column, where identifying information about the article is entered. This information can be anything that identifies a particular study for further review and citation in the research report. Author(s), year, and short title are typically sufficient. The second, or "methodology" column, provides brief information about the overall design of the study. Relevant types of information for this column are study type (cohort, case-control, ethnography, etc.), characteristics and size of the sample, data collection tools or measures, and analytic procedures used. The third, or "results" column, contains a brief summary of the most essential findings of the study. The results can be essential on two levels: (1) essential to the field, and (2) essential to the research focus at hand. It is important and ethical to include results that both support and refute the particular research hypothesis. The results of prior studies should help the researcher further refine the research question or hypothesis. Column four, or the "strengths" column, summarizes the strong features of the study (e.g., a cohort study that can demonstrate temporal order,

Table 6–1 Organization of Information from the Literature Review

Study	Methodology	Results	Strengths	Weaknesses
1. Bailey, 1992	Cohort 4,192 secondary school students Survey—3 waves Patterns of drug use Percentages Descriptive	Escalation of illicit substances is associated with continued use and initiation of illicit substances	Cohort Large N Transitions Careful analysis	No causal factors tested Self reports Attrition of heavier users Limited to SE US
2.				
3.				
4.				

random sampling technique, large sample size, validated tools). Ideally, some or most of these strengths will also characterize the study at hand. The last is the "weaknesses" column and includes notes on the limitations and potential biases of the study (e.g., limited external validity, low response rates, self-reported measures, insufficient tests for confounding). These limitations help to identify the launching point where the study at hand will contribute to the relevant field and body of knowledge.

WRITING THE LITERATURE REVIEW

A literature review can be the final goal of the report or a part of a larger research project. The typical format of the review is the introduction, body of the review, and conclusion. The introduction defines the topic and purpose and significance of the research study. Ideally, a sentence or two will indicate why the study is worth doing and the article worth reading. The body of the review summarizes the key features of the studies in some organized manner. The materials can be summarized by theme (i.e., general conclusions of the study), historical time (i.e., earlier to most recent studies), methodology (i.e., study design), target population, and so on. The appropriate organizational structure depends on the nature of the study at hand, but a common format is thematic. The body of the review includes a very brief summary and analysis of each work, including its importance to the overall topic, relationship to other referenced works, strengths, and weaknesses. The last component of literature review is the conclusion. Information included in this component covers the overall "lesson" learned from the studies, the authors' insights regarding the studies and general topic, and, most importantly, the specific contribution the present study will make to this group of studies or body of research.

It is appropriate to note, at this point, that prose from the article being reviewed should not be copied word for word without the use of quotation marks. In addition, direct quotations should be avoided, and conclusions should be stated in the words of the reviewer. Changing the verb tense or an adjective here and there does not count as using one's "own words." Plagiarism means presenting someone else's thoughts and ideas as if they were your own. This is a serious ethical violation that can and should result in punitive action.

Thematic Organization in the Body of the Review

Ideally, through the note-taking process, a conceptual picture will emerge and indicate meaningful themes for grouping studies based on similar results, designs, and/or conclusions. There are many specific methods for identifying themes. These include literature maps, spiderweb formats, outline formats, and conceptual trees. Below is an example of an outline format for reviewing literature focusing on Type 2 diabetes in children and adolescents. This literature review will present information on a general description of epidemiology, diagnosis, associated factors, treatment, and diabetes control. Sociodemographic, biomedical, and self-care behaviors as they relate to diabetes control will also be included.

Example outline:

I. Diabetes mellitus

II. Type 2 diabetes in children and adolescents

    A. Epidemiology
    B. Diagnosis
    C. Associated factors

        1. Relationship to obesity
        2. Other risk factors: puberty, ethnicity, gender, hypertension, metabolic syndrome

    D. Treatment of Type 2 diabetes in children and adolescents

III. Assessment of control in diabetes

    A. Definition of control
    B. Glycemic control
    C. Lipid management

IV. Determinants of diabetes control

    A. Sociodemographic factors
    B. Biomedical factors
    C. Self-care behaviors

        1. Medications
        2. Home diabetes status monitoring
        3. Exercise
        4. Diet
        5. Weight control
        6. Education

Summarizing the Major Themes

At this point, writing can begin. Using the outline or other organizational format, elements from the notes summary are converted to prose. For example, for each heading or subheading identified in the outline, relevant results or conclusions are summarized. A full summary for each study is provided in the study-by-study review of literature, and a brief summary of key results is included in the thematic literature review.

In a study-by-study review of literature, the author provides a detailed summary of each study under the specified theme. The detailed summary includes information on the research question addressed, methodology used, and findings of the study. This often requires a paragraph for each study. In this style of review, the author links similar studies (studies that fit under the same theme) using transitional sentences. The study-by-study style of literature review is used typically in term papers and theses or dissertations (Clark & Creswell, 2010). The following passage is an example of prose using this writing style:

> Data assessment from National Health and Nutrition Examination Survey (NHANES) III demonstrated that among 2,867 individuals aged 12–19 years between 1988 and 1994, 13 of those sampled had diabetes (Fagot-Campagna, Saadinem, Flegal, et al., 2001). Of these 13, 9 were based on insulin treatment and 2 on treatment with oral agents, and 2 on elevated fasting or random blood glucose levels. National prevalence estimates for all types of diabetes of 4.1 per 1,000 in this age group were hence calculated (Fagot-Campagna et al., 2001).

On the other hand, the thematic review of literature focuses on a theme and, in a succinct manner, cites multiple studies to document important findings under each theme. When using this method of literature review, authors mainly discuss the main findings or results from the literature rather than presenting details of every single study. Often authors report a particular finding and cite multiple references in parentheses. In this style, the same theme or findings have been reported by multiple studies (Clark & Creswell, 2010). This style of literature review is used in journal articles. An example of this style follows:

> Case studies in Ohio, South Carolina, and a few other states have shown increasing percentages of incident pediatric cases of diagnosed diabetes, with fewer than 4% reported before the 1990s and up to 45% in recent studies (Fagot-Campagna et al., 2001; Pinhas-Hamiel, Dolan, Daniels, et al., 1996). Those believed to be at greatest risk are minority children (Native, African, and Mexican-Americans) who are obese, inactive, and genetically predisposed to the development of Type 2 diabetes (Dabelea, Pettitt, Jones, et al., 1999).

Systematic review is another form of literature review that involves in-depth literature review to address a specific research question. The emphasis is on finding all relevant studies and assessing the study design and methodology employed. Systematic reviews strive to provide detailed, unbiased summaries of existing research in the area of interest. Systematic reviews are rigorous and follow a set of criteria. Some of the important characteristics of systematic review are clearly stated objectives and eligibility criteria for studies; explicit, reproducible methodology; systematic search that attempts to identify all studies that meet the eligibility criteria; assessment of the validity of the findings of all included studies; and systematic presentation and synthesis of the findings of the studies (Cook, Sackett, & Spitzer, 1995; Crombie & Davis, 2009; Higgins & Green, 2011).

In evidence-based public health, systematic reviews provide a statistical estimate of the net benefit of all the studies included in the review. This approach is called meta-analysis. One of the major benefits of meta-analysis (if a rigorous systematic review is conducted) is that it presents a systematic synthesis of literature and hence reduces the bias that could occur when conducting a narrative literature review. Meta-analysis usually combines results from many trials that attempt to answer similar questions; this provides more power to detect even small differences. A well conducted systematic review is the most essential step for a good meta-analysis. If the review is not conducted systematically or is not complete, then the quantitative estimate that meta-analysis provides is not precise enough. The search strategies used for meta-analysis should be comprehensive, and several electronic databases like MEDLINE and Cochrane Central Register of Controlled Trials are used to review articles. Very strict guidelines for inclusion and exclusion of literature articles are used. Once all the relevant studies have been identified, only the well conducted studies should be included in the review (based on the guidelines or checklist established). The results of meta-analysis are usually presented as a ratio of the frequency of the events in the intervention group to that of the control group (Crombie & Davis, 2009).

Though meta-analysis offers a systematic and quantitative approach to literature review, there can be flaws in analytic approach. Some of the major contributors to flaws in meta-analysis are (1) incomplete literature searches, (2) the inclusion of studies that did not completely meet rigorous inclusion criteria and may be of insufficient quality, and (3) the use of inappropriate or weak statistical methods to interpret the findings (Crombie & Davis, 2009). **Table 6–2** lists the steps involved in meta-analyses and a brief explanation of each step.

Cochrane Reviews, which are published in the Cochrane Database of Systematic Reviews, are an example of systematic reviews (meta-analyses). They serve as a good source for developing background information on a research topic. These systematic reviews help identify, appraise, and synthesize research-based evidence and present it in an accessible format.

Table 6–2 Steps Involved in Conducting Meta-Analyses

Steps	Brief description
Step 1: Location of studies	Comprehensive search strategy needs to be developed that targets several databases. A checklist should be developed with inclusion and exclusion criteria (e.g., select only studies with randomized clinical trials and so on).
Step 2: Quality assessment	Follow clear and objective criteria for evaluating studies based on quality. There are a number of scales available for assessing the quality of studies. Sensitivity analysis is also used to weed out the studies. Sensitivity analysis helps explore the effect of excluding various categories of studies and also helps interpret how consistent the results are across selected groups (age group, patient population, etc.).
Step 3: Calculating effect sizes	Effect sizes for a meta-analysis are summarized as the ratio of frequency of events in the intervention to that in the control group. Odds ratio and relative risk (risk ratio) are the two most common measures of effect size.
Step 4: Checking for publication bias	Publication bias is a key issue in meta-analysis. Clinical trials that exhibit a positive effect are more likely to be published than trials that demonstrate a negative effect. Funnel plot are used to display the presence of publication bias. These plots display studies included in the meta-analysis in a plot of effect size against sample size. If the resulting funnel plot is asymmetric, it means that some trials (usually the small trial showing no impact) might have been missed.
Step 5: Presenting the results	Forest plot: This is one of the most commonly used methods of presenting results from meta-analysis. This plot presents findings from each individual study as a small square or triangle. If the squares are on the left side of the neutral line (= 1), they indicate a positive impact of the treatment. If the squares are on the right side, this indicates that the treatment is less effective.

Study or Subgroup	Risk Ratio IV, Random, 95% CI	Year	Risk Ratio IV, Random, 95% CI
Coronary Heart Disease			
Shekelle et al. (17)	1.11 [0.91, 1.36]	1981	
McGee et al. (9)	0.66 [0.67, 1.12]	1984	
Kusni et al. (13)	1.33 [0.95, 1.87]	1985	
Posner et al. (16)	0.92 [0.68, 1.24]	1991	
Goldbount et al. (35)	0.86 [0.58, 1.35]	1993	
Fehlly et al. (28)	1.57 [0.56, 4.42]	1994	
Ascherio et al. (4)	1.11 [0.87, 1.42]	1996	
Esrey et al. (6)	0.97 [0.80, 1.18]	1996	

Heterogeneity: One of the major concerns of meta-analysis is how to combine or integrate data from different studies. Cochiran's Q (a statistical test based on chi-square) and I^2 statistic are used to test the existence of heterogeneity. The presence or absence of heterogeneity influences the choice for method of analysis.

Source: Data from Crombie, I. K., & Davis, H. T. O. (2009). *What is meta-analysis?* (2nd ed.). Newmarket, Suffolk, UK: Hayward Medical Communications; Sterne, J. A. C., & Harbord, R. M. (2004). Funnel plots in meta-analysis. *The Stata Journal, 4*(2), 127–141.

Example: Meta-Analysis of Prospective Cohort Studies Evaluating the Association of Saturated Fat with Cardiovascular Disease

A reduction in dietary saturated fat is believed to improve cardiovascular health by reducing the risk of coronary heart disease (CHD). To test this assumption, a meta-analysis was conducted to summarize evidence related to the association between dietary saturated fat with risk of coronary heart disease, stroke, and cardiovascular disease (CVD) (Siri-Tarino, Sun, Hu, et al., 2010). In this study, the investigators independently conducted systematic literature searches of two databases by using a set of search terms. The study used both within-study and between-study variability to calculate pooled relative risks (RR) across studies for the association between dietary saturated fat and CHD risk. The RR values provided no support for this association. Further analysis also showed that studies demonstrating significant associations were more likely to get published. The general conclusion of the meta-analysis is that there is no demonstrated association between reduced intake of dietary saturated fat and CHD risks, and a publication bias appears to be present in that studies showing significant relationships were more likely to get published.

Citations and References

Regardless of the purpose of the review, citations must be included in the paper. Credit should be given to authors, and statements made in the text should be supported with their source. There are several different styles of citation. The two most common styles are the American Psychological Association's style (APA style) and the American Medical Association's style (AMA style). Style manuals are available online to provide the guidelines for citing references. The choice of the citation style is determined by the teacher for class projects, by the college for professional degree thesis or dissertation, and by the journals for publishing research articles.

Citations are embedded within the text, and references are listed at the end of the report. Citations are indicated either by author last name(s) and year in parentheses or by numbers indicating the order in which they are cited. Numbers can be superscript, in brackets, and so on. The format for references at the end of the text varies widely by style. The information included typically includes authors' last names, first names or initials, year, journal or book title, volume and issue numbers, book edition, page numbers, and more (Clark & Creswell, 2010). **Table 6–3** presents some examples of AMA and APA styles of references. Before writing the research report, the required reference style should be noted and followed. Before submission, the style should be confirmed and proofread.

Managing references is a complicated task. Formatting references based on the wide variety of available citation styles can be very tedious and time consuming; therefore, using a reference management tool is essential. Using bibliographic or reference management software such as RefWorks, EndNote, Pages, or Reference

Table 6–3 Comparison of AMA and APA Styles of Referencing

Type of reference	AMA style	APA style
Books	Fitzgerald PA. *Handbook of Clinical Endocrinology*. 2nd ed. Norwalk, CT: Appleton & Lange; 1992.	Fitzgerald, P. A. (1992). *Handbook of clinical endocrinology*. Norwalk, CT: Appleton & Lange.
Article, single author	Ziegler TR. Glutamine supplementation in cancer patients receiving bone marrow transplantation and high dose chemotherapy. *J Nutr.* 2001;131(9): 2578B–2884B.	Ziegler, T. R. (2001). Glutamine supplementation in cancer patients receiving bone marrow transplantation and high dose chemotherapy. *Journal of Nutrition, 131*(9), 2578S–2584S.
Article, two to three authors	Mehl ML, Kyles AE. Ureteroureterostomy after proximal ureteric injury during an ovariohysterectomy in a dog. *Veterinary Record.* 2003;153(15):469–470.	Mehl, M. L., & Kyles, A. E. (2003). Ureteroureterostomy after proximal ureteric injury during an ovariohysterectomy in a dog. *Veterinary Record, 153*(15), 469–470.
Article, more than three authors	Nguyen NP, Moltz CC, Frank C, et al. Dysphagia following chemoradiation for locally advanced head and neck cancer. *Annals of Oncology.* 2004;15(3):383–388.	APA uses the same format for one to seven authors: Nguyen, N. P., Moltz, C. C., Frank, C., Vos, P., Smith, H. J., Karlsson, U., & Dutta, S. (2004). Dysphagia following chemoradiation for locally advanced head and neck cancer. *Annals of Oncology, 15*(3), 383–388. If more than seven authors: Nguyen, N. P., Moltz, C. C., Frank, C., Vos, P., Smith, H. J., Karlsson, U., . . . Dutta, S. (2004). Dysphagia following chemoradiation for locally advanced head and neck cancer. *Annals of Oncology, 15*(3), 383–388.

Manager, just to name a few, is very helpful to keep track of the references included in the literature review and to record them in the appropriate style. The choice of which software to use depends on what is available at your university or library. These tools help organize, search and sort, facilitate data storage, and also produce formatted citations. You can use these reference management tools to conduct searches as well as store the information on all search fields for each reference obtained during the literature search. These tools are developed to interface with word processing software to help organize and format references in a desired citation style. Formatting citations is one of the biggest advantages of using these reference management tools. If possible, try to avoid hand entering each citation due to the potential for error using this method.

CONCLUSION

The literature review serves several purposes in the research process. First, meaningful reviews of relevant studies help refine the research question or hypothesis and indicate the potential contributions the present study can make. Second, factual statements made in the text are supported. Third, details about the present study design are suggested or influenced. Finally, the significance of the study is defined. Some key tips for preparing an effective review are: (1) make it reasonably exhaustive, (2) include only relevant studies, (3) use recent studies as appropriate, (4) analyze as well as summarize the studies, (5) organize the summary in some meaningful way, typically by themes, and (6) emphasize the path from results of prior studies to the potential contribution of the present study.

VOCABULARY

Databases	Primary source	Systematic review
Heterogeneity	Publication bias	Thematic review
Keywords	Secondary source	
Meta-analysis	Study-by-study review	

STUDY QUESTIONS AND EXERCISES

1. What are the major sources of information for conducting a literature review?
2. State the important steps in filtering research.
3. Describe the process of organizing the summary of studies.
4. List two to three search terms or keywords you would use for research on the following scenarios:
   a. You are conducting a literature review on injury-related deaths. You are interested in comparing the numbers of unintentional and intentional deaths.
   b. You are interested in studying the influence of socioeconomic status and ethnic background on higher rates of obesity and cardiovascular risk factors.
5. Prepare a topic outline for the relevant literature review for your particular study or for a hypothetical study of "Obesity and Colorectal Cancer."

REFERENCES

Chatburn, R. L. (2011). *Handbook for health care research* (2nd ed.). Sudbury, MA: Jones & Bartlett.

Clark, V. L. P., & Creswell, J. W. (2010). *Understanding research: A consumer's guide*. Upper Saddle River, NJ: Pearson Education.

Cook, D. J., Sackett, D. L., & Spitzer, W. O. (1995). Methodologic guidelines for systematic reviews of randomized control trials in health care from the Potsdam Consultation on Meta-Analysis. *Journal of Clinical Epidemiology, 48*(1), 167–171.

Crombie, I. K., & Davis, H. T. O. (2009). *What is meta-analysis* (2nd ed.). Newmarket, Suffolk, UK: Hayward Medical Communications.

Dabelea, D., Pettitt, D. J., Jones, K. L., & Arslanian, S. A. (1999). Type 2 diabetes in minority children and adolescents: An emerging problem. *Endocrinology Metabolism Clinical of North America, 28*, 709–729.

Fagot-Campagna, A., Saadinem, J. B., Flegal, K. M., Beckles, G. L. (2001). Diabetes, impaired fasting glucose, and elevated HbA1c in US adolescents: The Third National Health and Nutrition Examination Survey. *Diabetes Care, 24*, 834–837.

Higgins, J. P. T., & Green, S. (Eds.). (2011). *Cochrane handbook for systematic reviews of interventions,* Version 5.1.0 [updated March 2011]. The Cochrane Collaboration. Retrieved February 5, 2012, from www.cochrane-handbook.org.

Johnson, B., & Christensen, L. (2008). *Educational research: Quantitative, qualitative, and mixed approaches* (2nd ed.). Thousand Oaks, CA: Sage Publications.

McMillan, J. H. (2008). *Educational research: fundamentals for the consumer* (5th ed.). Boston, MA: Pearson Education.

Pinhas-Hamiel, O. M., Dolan, L. M., Daniels, S. R., Standiford, D., Khoury, P. R., & Zeitler, P. (1996). Increased incidence of non-insulin dependent diabetes mellitus among adolescents. *The Journal of Pediatrics, 128*(5), 608–615.

Siri-Tarino, P. W., Sun, Q., Hu, F. B., & Krauss, R. M. (2010). Meta-analysis of prospective cohort studies evaluating the association of saturated fat with cardiovascular disease. *American Journal of Clinical Nutrition, 91*(3), 535–546.

CHAPTER 7

Obtaining Subjects

LEARNING OBJECTIVES

By the end of this chapter the reader will be able to:

- Determine the valid connection between the study sample, study population, and theoretical population.
- Identify and assemble appropriate sampling frames.
- Select samples using appropriate sampling methods.
- Recruit and retain study participants.
- Maximize internal and external validity.
- Calculate the required sample sizes.

CHAPTER OUTLINE

Have you seen "Crazy Curt" with the dragon tattoo the length of his arm and the eyebrow piercings? If you see him, tell him to come in for his follow-up.

—Research Assistant for a Study of Young
Injection Drug Users in Chicago

INTRODUCTION

This level of detail known about "Crazy Curt" (including that this is his "street name") illustrates the time, effort, thought, and forethought needed to recruit and, in this case, retain study participants. Successful specific recruitment and retention techniques depend on the focus, design, and target population of the study. In this chapter, we talk about techniques to obtain subjects for studies with more than 10 subjects (i.e., beyond case studies and series) and with the individual as the unit of analysis (i.e., excluding ecologic and community trials). The relevant study designs, then, are cross-sectional, case-control, cohort, and experimental studies. Subject selection and recruitment should be conducted in such a way that the resulting sample is "representative" of the study target population. These are discussed in the next section.

TARGET/THEORETICAL POPULATION AND SAMPLE

In 2009, 8.7% of Americans age 12 years or older were using illegal drugs (Substance Abuse and Mental Health Services Administration [SAMHSA], 2010). How do we know this? Obviously, surveying all 281.4 million Americans (U.S. Census Bureau, 2002) about their drug use habits would be prohibitive, if not impossible, due to exorbitant costs in money and time. Instead, the National Survey on Drug Use and Health (NSDUH) selected and surveyed a sample of 67,870 persons to "represent" the millions of Americans. Reasonable assumptions were made and strict procedures were used to select this sample so that its representativeness was known.

In this example, the target or theoretical population was Americans age 12 years and older in 2009, and a sample of these were selected for analysis.

The relationship between the theoretical population and the sample is illustrated in **Figure 7–1**. In this figure, the sample is represented by houses because the sample was selected first by dwelling unit. The arrow from the U.S. map to the group of houses represents the sampling process. (More specific information about the sampling procedure is discussed shortly.) Analysis was then conducted on the sample of 67,870 persons, and the results of the analysis are said to represent the behavior of all Americans age 12 years or older. The assumption that the results of the sample represent those that we would find if we surveyed the entire population of Americans age 12 years or older is called generalization. Formally, generalizability is the degree to which study results are valid for members of the study population not included in the sample. The truth of this assumption depends on the rigor and appropriateness of the sampling procedure.

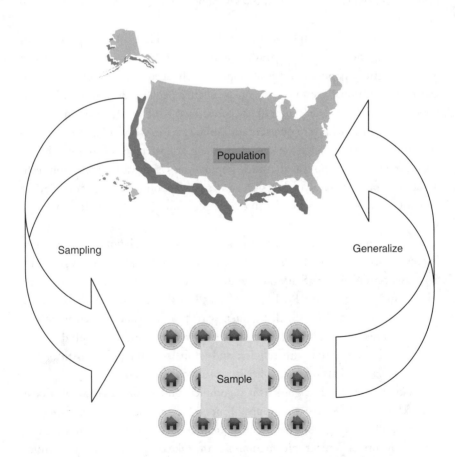

FIGURE 7–1 Connections Between Sample and Theoretical/Target Population

SAMPLE POPULATION AND SAMPLING FRAME

The valid or accurate connection between sampling and generalization sounds good in theory, but how is it accomplished in reality? Obviously, the investigator must have direct access to the population of interest. Typically, the group accessible to the investigator is a subset of the target population. The group is accessible through face-to-face contact or through the availability of reliable contact information. This group to whom researchers can make contact is called the sample population or study population. The list of their names and contact information is called the sampling frame. The sample of individuals actually included in the study is chosen in some fashion from the sampling frame. The relationships between the population, sampling frame, and sample are illustrated in **Figure 7–2**.

Staying with the example of the NSDUH (SAMHSA, 2010), the target or theoretical population, as previously stated, was all Americans age 12 years or older. The study population was all appropriately aged residents of households and noninstitutional group quarters (e.g., shelters, college dormitories, halfway houses) and civilians living on military bases. That is, all residents of households and noninstitutional group quarters and military bases who had addresses available to researchers through various sources (e.g., department of motor vehicles, tax records). This group was the study population. Using various selection techniques, a sampling frame of 178,013 addresses was compiled. Of these, 85,744 individuals were selected for the study sample, and 67,780 participated in the survey.

Other examples of theoretical populations, study populations, and sampling frames, respectively, are (1) hospital patients with gall bladder disease; gall bladder patients in New York State and California; gall bladder patients in one hospital each in New York City, Rochester, Albany, Buffalo, Los Angeles, Sacramento, San Francisco, and Bakersfield; (2) men with prostate cancer; men who have been diagnosed and treated; men in the cancer registry; and (3) morbidly obese adults; adults diagnosed with obesity; and adults scheduled for gastric bypass surgery at six hospitals that specialize in treatments for obesity.

A sampling frame is as good as it is complete and accurate. A sample drawn from a frame will be biased if groups of individuals in the study population are systematically missing from the frame or are more likely than others to have outdated or incorrect contact information. For the sake of sample validity, attention to accuracy and thoroughness in compiling the frame is essential. If necessary, the

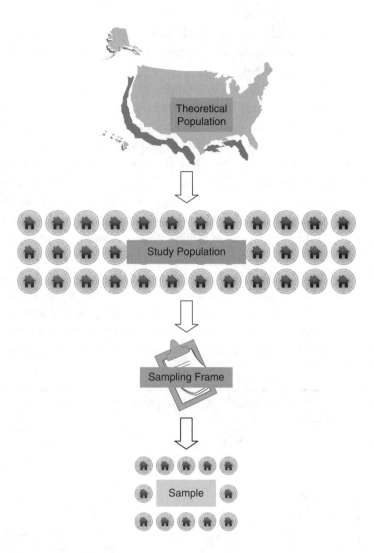

FIGURE 7–2 Sampling Process

study population may need to be limited by the availability of information for the frame. For example, the study population for NSDUH is limited to residents of households and noninstitutionalized group settings because contact information for homeless individuals who do not use shelters and are not institutionalized (e.g., mental institutions, nursing homes, correctional facilities) persons is unavailable or protected. When the study population is limited by the sampling frame, the generalizability of the sample to the theoretical population is also limited. This shortcoming should be acknowledged by study personnel in the interpretation of study results.

Not only does the benefit to sample validity justify the time and effort needed to construct a complete and correct sampling frame, but validity cannot be achieved if the wrong frame is accessed in the first place. The research question should drive the choice of sampling frames through both its substantive focus and its influence on study design. The links between research question, study design, and sampling frame are illustrated in **Table 7–1**. In each of the examples presented in Table 7–1, the sampling frames include identification or contact information for potential study participants. Sometimes the frames represent a region of the United States or are believed to be representative of the United States in general. In all cases, the characteristics of persons in the sampling frame are directly relevant to the research question.

There are two ways that a sample can be representative of the population. These are expressed as internal and external validity and are illustrated in **Figure 7–3**. Internal validity expresses how well the sample represents the study or sample population (the group available to the researchers). The more rigorous

Table 7–1 Link Between Research Question, Study Design, and Sampling Frame

Research question	Study design	Sampling frame
What are the causes and correlates of experimental versus continuing use of marijuana among middle school students in the southeast United States?	Prospective cohort	Homeroom lists of students in five middle schools in Wake County, NC
What are the risk factors for knee injuries among female teenage soccer players in the Midwest United States?	Case-control	Patient numbers of teenage female soccer players at three orthopedic clinics in Chicago and surrounding suburbs (one-third with knee injuries and two-thirds with other injuries)
What is the prevalence of neurological problems among residents living near natural gas wells?	Cross-sectional	Addresses of household residents in 50 rural areas in the PA Marcellus Shale region
Is synthetic tissue grafting as effective as biological tissue grafting in treating dental gum recession?	Randomized controlled trial	Patient numbers of adults seeking treatment for gum recession (with otherwise healthy gums) in three large dental practices in St. Louis, MO

and controlled the sampling method, the greater the internal validity. External validity indicates how well the sample represents the target population. It should be emphasized that if a sample does not have internal validity, then it could not possibly have external validity. If it does not represent the sample population, then it could not represent the target population. This level of validity depends not only on the quality of the sampling method, but also on the selection of the sample population and the choice and compilation of the sampling frame.

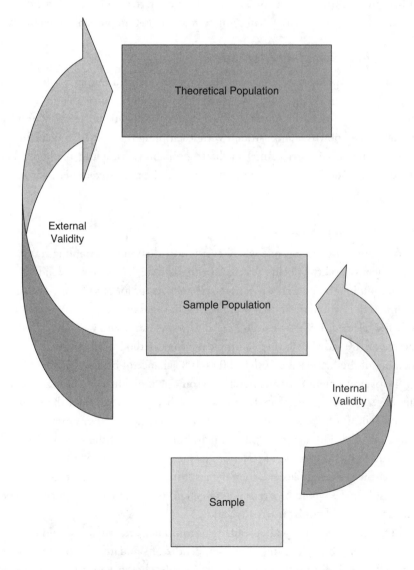

FIGURE 7–3 Internal and External Validity

SAMPLING METHODS

With a complete and accurate sampling frame, subject selection can now begin. However, not all sampling methods are equal in their ability to select samples that are representative of the target population. Generally, probability samples are superior to non-probability samples in that the former can exert the most control over selection and can assign probability values of being selected for the study. When probabilities of selection are known, the internal and external validity of the sample can be evaluated. Sampling frames are used in probability methods.

Probability Sampling Methods

Probability sampling methods have the ability to assign a numeric value to the probability of any one person being chosen for the study. To be able to calculate the probability value, the number of potential participants in the study population must be known. Hence, studies with a sampling frame (with a quantifiable group of potential participants) facilitate probability sampling methods. The choice of method depends on research focus and the need to represent particular characteristics of the study population.

Simple Random Sample

A truly random sample is one where every individual in the sampling frame has the same probability of being selected for the sample. Say we have N individuals in our sampling frame, and we want to select n persons for our sample. Truly random selection would mean that every person in the frame has an n/N probability of being selected. If we have 1,000 persons in our frame and we want to select a sample of 100 individuals, then a simple random method would mean that every member of the frame has a 100/1,000 or 10% chance of being selected.

If, for any practical or theoretical reason, an individual in the frame actually has a greater or less than 10% chance of being selected, then the resulting sample will not be randomly selected in the strictest sense. For example, if our frame includes 500 men and 500 women, but, because of the way the frame is constructed or the method of selection, women really have a 15% and men have a 5% chance of being selected, then the resulting sample would be biased toward females. Females would be overrepresented and males underrepresented. Hence, the sample would not be internally valid.

In the days before the widespread use of computers, researchers would use random number tables often found in an appendix of standard statistics textbooks. This table includes numbers that are randomly chosen and randomly placed in the table. The investigator would then choose n numbers (without duplicating a number) by blindly pointing to a starting number in the table, then moving up or down or across or diagonally through the table until n unique numbers are chosen. Numbers are assigned to each member of the frame before selection begins, then the person assigned with the first number randomly selected from the random number table is chosen for the sample. Today, many random number generators are available in computer packages. Excel has such a generator called RAND. These programs are more commonly used for random selection in contemporary studies.

Other Random Selection Methods

Although the simple random sampling method is the ideal in terms of maximizing validity of the sample, sometimes this method is not possible or even appropriate. Other random selection methods are appropriate particularly when researchers wish to include sufficient numbers of persons with certain characteristics to formulate a group large enough to analyze with statistical methods. We will first discuss a random method that can be used when simple random sampling is not feasible.

Systematic random sampling can be used in situations where assigning numbers to sampling frame units is unwieldy. For example, say a researcher wants to estimate the prevalence of HIV in parts of Africa. She has boxes and boxes of 221,056 blood samples collected from health clinics across Sub-Sahara Africa, but only enough funding to conduct 2,000 Western Blot and Elisa tests. Therefore, she must take a sample of about 10% of the specimens. She has a list of patient identification numbers, but these are not unique nor in a consistent format. In addition, due to improper placement of specimens in boxes, some of the test tube labels were rendered unreadable. Consequently, she chooses to conduct a systematic random sampling. **Figure 7–4** illustrates this method.

Her sampling frame is now the test tubes themselves numbered with a consistent method within their storage boxes. Each box contained 100 samples. For a systematic sampling, the researcher needs to choose every kth tube where $k = N/n$. In this example $k = 221,056/2,000$ or 110.5. Hence, the researcher chose every 110th tube of blood. To determine where to begin this pattern of selection, the researcher randomly chose a number between 1 and 110. Say she chose 23, so the 23rd tube was her first selection. Next, she chose the 133rd (23 + 110) tube, then the 243rd tube and so on until she selected 2,000 samples. This method is called systematic random sampling, because units are chosen randomly, but in a systematic or patterned fashion.

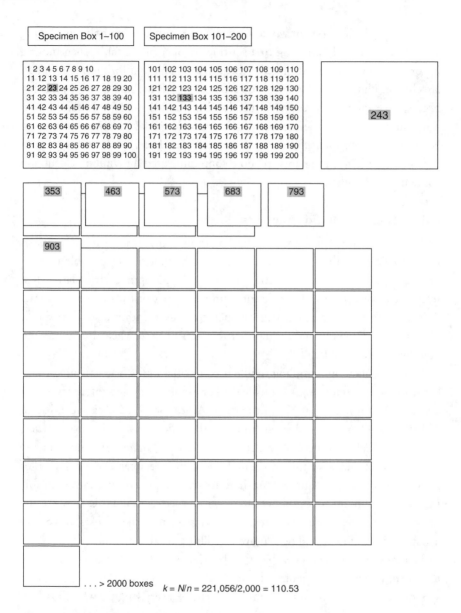

FIGURE 7–4 Example of Systematic Random Sampling

Stratified random sampling is another common random selection method. This method is used when researchers wish to include units with relatively rare characteristics in the sampling frame. In other words, they want to assign a greater than simply random probability of selecting units with particular characteristics. This is called over-sampling.

The NSDUH uses a stratified random sampling method for selecting Americans ages 12 years and older. First, eight states were designated as large sample states (e.g., California, New York, Illinois). Then states were stratified or grouped into 900 field interview regions (48 regions in each large sample state and 12 in each small sample state). Within each region, adjacent census blocks were combined to form area segments. Next, 96 segments per 900 regions were selected with probability proportionate to population size (i.e., segments with larger population sizes had greater probabilities of selection). Finally, eight segments within each region (out of the 96 segments per region) were chosen randomly for the study. The stratified method was used to assure the representation of households in areas with small populations.

Figure 7–5 illustrates a simpler example of stratified random sampling. In this hypothetical study, a randomized controlled trial is designed to test the efficacy of a supplemental medication to treat clinical depression. Due to past negative experiences with antidepressants among adolescents, study funders required that sufficient numbers of young people be included in the trial to support analyses by age group. (Appropriate pretests, parental consent procedures, and risk precautions were used.) Potential subjects were recruited by pharmacists' initial contact letters. The initial pool of 1,500 persons were stratified or grouped by age range, and subjects, whenever possible, were randomly selected within age strata. Nearly all (83%) of the young people were selected; 50% of the adult and middle-aged group were chosen; and 40% of the older adults were included. In the original pool of volunteers, 20% were in the younger group; 47% in the middle group; and 33% in the older group. After stratification and sampling, the study group proportions were 31% youth, 44% adults, and 25% older adults. Hence, young people were over-sampled, adults sampled nearly proportionate to the original group size, and older adults under-sampled.

Stratified samples in which strata are over- and under-sampled are called disproportionate stratified samples. In other words, different sampling probabilities are used across strata. When estimates are made about population prevalence and other parameters in disproportionate samples, sampling weights must be applied to the estimates to adjust for differential sampling probabilities.* When strata have equal probabilities of selection, then the varying sizes of the strata will be represented proportionately. This type of stratified sample

---

*See Lee and Forthofer (2006) for a more detailed discussion about sampling weights.

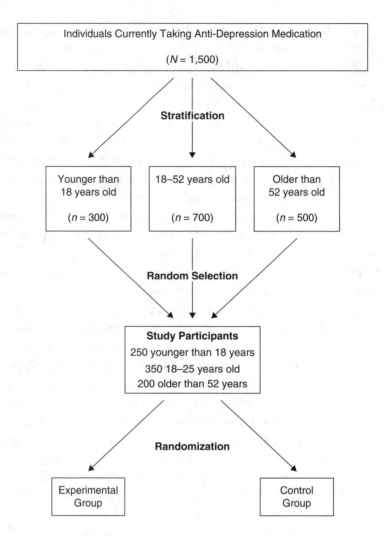

FIGURE 7–5 Example of Stratified Random Sampling

is call proportionate. Population estimates in proportionate samples do not require sampling weights.

These and other random sampling methods can be used in combination through two or more stages of sampling. This is multistage sampling. For example, a sampling frame can be separated into strata, and units can be systematically sampled from the strata. Simple random sampling is the ideal in terms of its ability to minimize sampling or selection bias. Other random methods may also be used alone or in combination depending on the goals of the study and the characteristics of the sampling frame.

Nonprobability Sampling Methods

In a large proportion of epidemiologic studies, probability sampling methods are not possible because no sampling frame is available. Imagine compiling a list of homeless persons, illegal drug users, or sexually abused children. Lists of persons attending homeless shelters, drug treatment clinics, and hospital emergency rooms can be used, but the resulting samples will only represent a portion of the population of the homeless, drug users, or abused children. If the research questions require samples of homeless people living on the street or precariously housed, drug users who do not seek treatment, or abused children who have not sought medical care, then nonprobability sampling methods must be used. For these methods, the probability of selection of sample units is unknown. Hence, the representativeness of the theoretical or target sample is also unknown. Potential selection bias must be acknowledged when reporting the results of nonprobability samples.

Convenience Sampling

Members of convenience samples are those that are conveniently available to researchers, but are not selected from a sampling frame with any measurable representativeness. Convenience sampling is also called haphazard or accidental. Examples are subjects who respond to study advertisements, an investigator's college class of students, voters exiting polling centers, or attendees at a health fair. A mistake often made in studies using convenience samples is overreaching in terms of claiming or just assuming sample representativeness. In actuality, little can be known about the relevant characteristics of a target population or even study population in studies using convenience samples. Results can still be valuable, but they must be kept in perspective in terms of limited generalizability.

Purposive Sampling

In epidemiologic research, purposive sampling is the most common type of nonprobability sampling. Purposive sampling is sampling with a "purpose." The targets of this method have particular characteristics (e.g., middle-aged women with stage 1 breast cancer) directly related to the research question. Study subjects are identified through a method that does not use a sampling frame. For example, middle-aged women with stage 1 breast cancer can be recruited at breast cancer awareness events. Women who voluntarily acknowledge their cancer status would be asked at the event to participate in the study.

There are several variations of purposive sampling methods. The variations depend on the source of subjects, the nature of the required characteristics, and/ or the procedure for identifying potential participants. The purpose of expert sampling is to recruit subjects with a particular expertise related to the research question. Reasons to use this approach are to document experts' views on the topic of interest or to validate some aspect of a larger study. For example, a new or controversial measurement procedure or working definition can be evaluated by an expert sample.

Modal instance sampling would be used to elicit the "typical" response, opinion, or status of the hypothetical population, loosely defined because this is not a probability method. Potential subjects with the modal or most common status are usually defined as persons with relevant "average" characteristics—for example, the average age, race/ethnicity, and socioeconomic status of women with stage 1 breast cancer. On the other hand, heterogeneity sampling is used when a study needs to include a broad array of subject characteristics, not just the average. Finally, quota sampling is a method used to include an array of subject characteristics in predefined proportions. If the hypothetical breast cancer study requires 40% of the sample to be African American, then in a study of 100 subjects, qualified African American women will be recruited at the event until 40 are enrolled. When 40 are recruited, no more African American women will be approached to participate. As in stratified random sampling, the desired proportion can either reflect the actual proportion in the theoretical population (proportional) or, usually for analytic reasons, over- or under-represent the true proportions (disproportionate).

Snowball sampling is a particular technique to identify a purposive sample. A few individuals with the required characteristics are identified by some method, and then researchers ask them to recommend people they know with the required study criteria for study recruitment. The initial participants provide contact information to study personnel, who then contact the recommended persons and ask them to participate. Subjects in the resulting sample are likely to be very similar to each other and certainly not representative of a target population, but this method may be the only procedure available. This is particularly true for studies of hidden or relatively inaccessible populations, such as homeless persons who do not use shelters, illegal drug users not in treatment, or illegal immigrants.

A variation of the snowball sampling approach is respondent-driven sampling (RDS) (Heckathorn, 2011). Studies of injection drug users have used this technique to recruit study participants (Abdul-Quadar, Heckathorn, Sabin, et al., 2006; Magnani, Sabin, Saidel, et al., 2005). First, young injection drug users who used needle exchange were recruited to participate in the study. These initial participants are called "seeds." Seeds were then given recruitment coupons with information about the study and asked to give the coupons to young injection drug users they know. For each eligible person who enrolled in the study and had a coupon from the seed, the seed was paid a monetary incentive. The recruitment method then continued by giving the newly enrolled subject recruitment coupons, and so on. Each round of recruitment is called a generation—seeds being the first generation. Methodological research on RDS suggests that by a certain generation of recruitment (i.e., the fourth or fifth generation), the resulting sample is fairly representative of the assumed theoretical population.[*]

SAMPLE RECRUITMENT AND RETENTION

With the target population defined, the sample population and sampling frame identified and compiled, and the sample units selected, the next huge step is to make contact with persons sampled and invite them to participate in the study. Recruitment is the point where the researcher's "best laid plans" are tested. This phase of research is essentially "marketing" the study. More specifically, the investigator must promote the study to the potential participants. Formally, promotion "is the communication link between sellers and buyers for the purpose of influencing, informing, or persuading a potential buyer's purchasing decision" (Boone & Kurtz, 2011).

Initial Contact

Like the consent form, the language and reading level of all recruitment materials should be appropriate for the potential study participants. Clarity and brevity are the ideal. Now, we begin with the "informing" component of promotion. Informing begins with the initial contact with potential subjects. Ideally, the method of contact will be similar to the method of data collection—in-person, traditional mail, telephone, or Internet. Initial contact can also be made through referrals by professionals, such as physicians, pharmacists, or therapists. Professional referrals are most appropriate for studies with direct benefits to subjects, but the referral should make it clear whether or not the professional is a stakeholder in the study. Proposed contact materials must be reviewed in the institutional review board's (IRB) initial study review. These include introduction

---

[*]See Heckathorn (1997) for a more detailed description of RDS and evidence of the representativeness of RDS samples.

letters and scripts for personal contacts and referrals. Brochures are often a user-friendly method for describing the study. Excerpts from the NSDUH introduction letter are presented in **Figure 7–6**. The introductory letter should communicate the "who, what, where, and when" of the study. In this example, the "who" is the Department of Health and Human Services (DHHS), Public Health Service, Research Triangle Institute (RTI), Assistant Project Officer, RTI Field Director, and toll-free contact number. The "what" is an interview about health-related issues in all segments of the American population and some preliminary screening questions. (This description is vague because the field interviewer is

LOGO   DEPARTMENT OF HEALTH AND HUMAN SERVICES   [ADDRESS]

_____, 2001

Dear Resident,

To better serve all aspects of the American population, the United States Department of Health and Human Services (DHHS), United States Public Health Service is conducting a national survey on health-related issues. Along with more than 200,000 other residences, your household was randomly selected for participation in the study. Research Triangle Institute (RTI) is under contract with DHHS to conduct the survey, and soon one of the professional field interviewers will be in your neighborhood to provide you with more information.

When the RTI representative arrives, please ask to see his or her personal identification card. (An example of the ID card is shown below.) He or she will ask a few preliminary questions, and then may ask one or possibly two members of your household to participate in a voluntary interview. It is also possible that, following the initial questions, no one from your household will be asked to participate. If any members of your household are selected for the interview and choose to participate, they will receive a cash payment of $_____ at the end of the interview in appreciation for their time.

Feel free to ask the RTI representative any questions you may have about the study. This survey is authorized by Section 505 of the Public Health Service Act. The confidentiality of the information collected is protected under Section 501 of the Public Health Service Act. The information collected is confidential and will only be used for research and analysis and cannot be used for any other purpose. This letter is addressed to "Resident" because the initial selection is made by address, and we are unaware of your name.

Your help is extremely important to the success of this study, and we thank you in advance for your cooperation.

Sincerely yours,

[SIGNATURE]

[NAME]
Assistant Project Officer, DHHS   [PICTURE IDENTIFICATION BADGE]

[SIGNATURE]

[NAME]
National Field Director, RTI
[TOLL-FREE NUMBER]   _____
                                Assigned Field Representative

FIGURE 7–6 Example of an Introduction Letter

empowered to describe, in person, the sensitive topic of the survey.) The "where" is the individual's place of residence. The "when" is soon relative to the date of the letter, which is probably vague for practical reasons.

The promotional aspects of the letter are intended to persuade the potential participants to answer the field interviewer's questions and possibly participate in the study. To this end, the letter emphasizes the importance and legitimacy of the study. The study is intended "to better serve all aspects of the American population." The survey is "authorized by Section 505 of the Public Health Service Act." Potential respondents' "help is extremely important to the success of the study." Individuals' time and effort is so important to the study that they will be given a cash payment. The legitimacy of the study is illustrated by using DHHS letterhead, listing the legal authorizations, presenting signatures of the project officer and field director, including a picture of the identification badge, and providing a phone number for verification. Confidentiality of subjects' data is assured by naming Section 501, and anonymity at this point in the study is highlighted.

The potential respondent is left to weigh his or her costs and benefits of participation. Costs that this may be a scam, that their time will be wasted, and that their personal information will be made public are addressed in the letter. Benefits to the participant are contributing to something important to better serve society and a cash payment to compensate for their time (although not from the point of view of the IRB). Hopefully, at this point, the potential subject is interested and comfortable enough to interact with the field interviewer when they knock on the front door. This interaction will be the final effort to recruit the respondent, and the complete nature of the study will be revealed.

Incentives to Participate

Cash incentives are not considered benefits in human subject reviews. However, they can often mean the difference between participation and nonparticipation in a study. In 2002, the NSDUH (then called the National Household Survey on Drug Abuse—the name of the study has since been changed to increase response rates) conducted a study on the effects of incentives on response rates (Eyerman, Odom, Wu, et al., 2002). They compared the rates for three groups of potential respondents: (1) those offered no cash incentive, (2) those offered $20, and (3) those offered $40. They found that the greater the incentive amount, the greater the response: (1) 69.2%, (2) 78.8%, and (3) 83.3% response, respectively. Generally, incentives (cash or service) are a powerful motivator in promoting the study.

However, the value of the incentive should not be so great as to be an undue influence to participate. The line between influential and coercive depends on the target population, the incentive, and the study risks. This line is evaluated by the IRB. A related ethical issue involving incentives is offering cash to populations who are likely to use the money for harmful purposes. Is the researcher causing more harm to the subject by offering a cash incentive? Illegal drug users are an obvious example of such a population. Nonpublished, largely anecdotal information from studies of injection drug users in Chicago indicated that potential subjects offered gift certificates as study incentives typically sold the certificates for less-than-face value and used the proceeds to buy drugs. Offering no incentives led to virtually no response. Consequently, the studies commenced offering cash incentives and were consistently asked to justify these to funders and IRB reviews. There is no correct answer as to the suitability of offering cash incentives to such populations, but this dilemma illustrates the conflict between societal good (i.e., obtaining information that may help prevent injection drug use in the future) and harm (i.e., enabling immediate drug use).

Screening

For purposive sampling and for possibly most probability-based studies, the targeted characteristics of potential participants need to be assessed or verified. For case-control and randomized controlled trials, precise screening for inclusionary and exclusionary criteria is essential. Usually, the appropriate time for screening is when the potential subject expresses a willingness to participate. The screening process should be scripted so that all members of the study team will be using identical screening criteria. **Figure 7–7** presents excerpts of the script for screening in the NSDUH study.

During the initial contact, potential subjects should be told that they may not be eligible to participate if they do not have certain characteristics. Note in the letter presented in Figure 7–7 that residents are told that the RTI field interviewer "will ask a few preliminary questions." The letter goes on to inform residents that "it is possible, following the initial questions, no one from your household will be asked to participate." As in all stages of the study involving human subjects, participants should be informed about everything they will experience, even in the screening process.

Note how the script gives precise wording for the screening questions so that all interviewers will conduct the screening in the same exact way. The screening criteria for this study are simple—the respondent must live most of the time at the address and must be age 12 years or older. Recall that the target population

---

Excerpts from NSDUH Screening Script

Hello, my name is [*Field Interviewer Name*] with the Research Triangle Institute in North Carolina. We are conducting a nationwide study sponsored by the U.S. Public Health Service.

You should have received a letter explaining the study.

IF NOT, HAND THE PERSON A COPY OF THE LETTER

First, let me just verify, do you live here?

IF NOT OBVIOUS:

And are you 18 or older?

I just need to verify this address.

EDIT ADDRESS IF INCORRECT

[*Have/Will*] you or anyone else [*lived/live*] here for most of the time during the months of [CURRENT QUARTER]?

[Including yourself], how many people in this household [*lived/will live*] here most of the time during the months of [CURRENT QUARTER]?

ENTER NUMBER 1–20

Of these [TOTAL NUMBER OF RESIDENTS], how many are age 12 or older?

Next, I'll ask a few questions about the people who live here. Let's start with the person or one of the persons living here who owns or rents this home. We'll refer to this person as the householder.

Please tell me the age of this person at his or her last birthday. OR Please tell me your age at your last birthday.

[And so on for each eligible household member.]

FIGURE 7–7 Examples of Screening Questions

Source: Office of Applied Studies. (2009). National survey on drug use and health [Computer file]. ICPSR29621-v2. Ann Arbor, MI: Inter-University Consortium for Political and Social Research [distributor], 2012-02-10. doi:10.3886/ICPSR29621.v2

for the study is household residents age 12 years or older. The general research question is: "What is the prevalence of illicit drug use among U.S. residents age 12 years and older?" **Table 7–2** presents other examples of research questions and a relevant screening process. The screening processes are intended to determine the relevant inclusionary and exclusionary criteria to represent the target population and, sometimes, for practical reasons in the successful conduct of the study. For example, the trial testing the effectiveness of the oral gum graft limited the sample to those without ongoing risk factors for further

Table 7–2 Examples of Research Questions and Relevant Screening Process

Research Question	Screening Process
What is the incidence of hepatitis C virus (HCV) among injection drug users in Chicago?	Screen for injection drug use by asking questions about the injection process and examining for needle marks. Screen for HCV with blood test. Exclude those who do not inject drugs and those who test positive for HCV.
Are adults who participated in elite club sports as children more likely than those who did not participate in high-level sports to require knee eplacement surgery?	Screen the medical records (after obtaining consent) of orthopedic patients. Select those who had knee replacement surgery in the past 12 months (cases). Select those who did and do not need knee replacement surgery but have a variety of chronic knee problems (controls). Exclude all patients with other types of problems.
Are synthetic grafts as successful as biological grafts for patients needing dental gum surgery?	Screen the dental records (after obtaining consent) of periodontic patients. Choose patients age 40 years and older scheduled for gingival grafting 2 weeks or longer in the future. Exclude those with ongoing risk factors such as uncorrected severe tooth crowding, active eating disorder, current use of chewing tobacco, lip or tongue piercing, and uncontrollable bruxism. Exclusion criteria are evaluated through record review and screening interviews with potential subjects.
What is the prevalence of endocrine disruption among individuals who consume well water in areas with a history of drilling for natural gas?	Screen all persons living within 15 miles of a gas drill initiated at least 5 years ago. Select residents who use well water for at least 50% of their water needs (e.g., drinking, washing dishes, bathing, brushing teeth).

gum recession, so that the potential effectiveness will not be compromised by extraneous factors. Careful thought should be given to the utility of screening criteria so that the final sample best represents the target population, nothing more and nothing less.

The value of cohort and experimental studies depends on subject retention between baseline and follow-up, between pretest and posttest, and possibly longer. There are two aspects to the importance of retention. First, as discussed in more detail at the end of this chapter, the ability to find statistically significant results depends largely on sample size. If a cohort or experimental study loses so many subjects by follow-up that this ability is compromised, then the entire study is considerably weakened. Second, if the subjects lost to follow-up are similar to each other and different from those retained in some way that may affect the relationship between exposure and outcome, then the sample is significantly biased.

So, how can we maximize subject retention? Specific methods depend on the data collection methods and characteristics of the study population. Two general pieces of advice are (1) to be creative, and (2) to have multiple ways to maintain contact with subjects. As for initial recruitment, ongoing promotion of the study, including subject incentives, is vital to retention. In fact, long-term studies sometimes increase the incentive and offer bonuses with each subsequent follow-up. Again, the incentive should not increase to a value that is unduly influential.

Methods to find "Crazy Curt," as mentioned in the introduction of this chapter, are an example of creativity in contact methods specific to the characteristics of the study population. Many injection drug users spend some time living on the street or in precarious housing. Young users are often kicked out of their parents' homes. Keeping record of "street names," identifying characteristics, and "running buddies" or friends helps to locate subjects with no stable address or telephone number through their social or casual networks. In addition, users are often in and out of the local jail. Because inmates can be searched in jail databases using their identification numbers but not names, record-keeping of jail identification numbers is also important for maintaining contact.

Even if the subject has a stable address and phone number, one of each is not enough. Depending on the specific characteristics of the population, contact information for relatives, friends, and neighbors can be useful. One suggestion is to record the contact information for one or two people who "would always know how to contact" the subject. Of course, work or school information should also be recorded if available. Knowledge about subjects' affiliations with institutions that keep contact records themselves (e.g., payroll information, alumni lists) can be very helpful. Necessary releases of information may need to be obtained from subjects during baseline data collection.

Over the course of the study, the contact information should be checked or verified to see if it is still valid. Verification methods include Internet searches on People-Finder and social network sites, record searches, and mail and telephone calls. Reminder postcards can be mailed, emails sent, and calls made to alert subjects to upcoming follow-ups. Birthday and holiday cards can be mailed to see if they are returned undeliverable. Again, creativity should be used in light of the specific characteristics of the study population.

A final component of subject retention is persistence. Numerous pieces of mail, emails, and phone calls may be necessary to locate and contact subjects for follow-up. The study protocol should include detailed and thoughtful procedures for follow-up contacts. A balance must be struck between effectiveness and harassment. If a subject declines after moderate persuasion, then research staff should take "no" for an answer. At this point, it is helpful to try to collect information from the subject about why he or she does not want to continue with the study. Such information is helpful in assessing bias in attrition, as well as study procedures that are not generally acceptable to subjects. An example of a reasonable protocol for an in-person follow-up is to send a reminder postcard, up to four reminder calls and/or emails, and possibly a field staff visit to the home address, if practical.

Unless it compromises the validity of the sample, potential subjects can be screened and excluded at baseline if they have plans to move away or be sent away (e.g., military, incarcerated) during the study period. Some combination of these retention methods is likely appropriate for most types of studies. Creativity, practicality, study resources, and respect for subjects all play a role in the design of the retention procedures. Much effort should be spent designing and following these procedures due to the serious threat to sample validity from significant loss of baseline subjects.

INTERNAL AND EXTERNAL VALIDITY

A scientifically rigorous study is one that addresses actual and potential threats to validity. Threats to internal and external validity are relevant to sample selection and retention. A direct threat to external validity is a mistaken conceptualization of the study population and the construction of an inappropriate sampling frame. External generalizability is limited by the available sample population. Without internal validity, there can be no external validity. If the sample does not represent the study population, it is impossible for it to represent the target or theoretical population. **Table 7–3** describes types of biases that threaten internal and external validity.

Selection, nonresponse, and attrition biases are all direct threats to internal validity. Selection bias is systematic error committed when sampling from the sampling frame. If a random procedure is planned and claimed but is not conducted properly, then selection bias may be the result. Simply put, if it is assumed that each unit has an equal probability of selection, but the assumption is untrue for some reason, then the sample is biased. If women actually have a 0.8 probability and men a 0.2 probability of selection, then the resulting sample will be biased toward women. Actual probabilities of selection should be evaluated and acknowledged in discussions of results in the context of generalizability.

Nonresponse bias occurs if selected subjects who consent to participate in the study are systematically different in a way that may affect results from

Table 7–3 Potential Biases in the Process of Obtaining Subjects

Source of bias	Explanation	Example
Sample selection	Potential subjects sampled from the study population are systematically different from those not sampled.	If patients with knee replacement surgery are selected primarily from orthopedic practices that specialize in sports medicine then the strength of the relationship between childhood participation in elite sports and knee replacement surgery will be overestimated (reasonably assuming the adults who were serious athletes as children are likely to be athletic as adults).
Nonresponse	Selected potential subjects who participate in the study are systematically different from those who do not agree to participate.	Residents who reside near natural gas wells and are feeling ill are more likely to participate in a study of endocrine disruption than are residents who live near wells but are not feeling ill. This type of bias will result in an overestimation of the prevalence of endocrine disruption in this population.
Attrition	Subjects who participated in the baseline measurement in cohort and experimental studies **and** who also participated in subsequent follow-up measures are systematically different from baseline subjects who were lost to follow-up measurements.	If injection drug users who are homeless and very heavy users of multiple types of drugs at baseline are more likely than others to be lost to follow-up, then the incidence of HCV will likely be underestimated.

selected persons who do not participate. For example, the NSDUH study has traditionally had a lower response rate (the percentage who participate out of total who were asked to participate) for African American persons compared to Caucasians and other races/ethnicities. As a result of the Tuskegee Syphilis Study and for other reasons, African Americans are more likely than Caucasians to be distrustful of research. The result is a sample that is biased toward Caucasians. To the extent that this type of nonresponse bias cannot be avoided, it should be measured by comparing the characteristics of sampled persons who responded to the characteristics of those who refused or were unavailable. Such biases should be reported in publications of results. Failing to do so is a violation of research ethics in reporting and interpreting study results. As a general rule of thumb, a response rate of 80% is considered high enough to have minimized adequately nonresponse bias. If lower rates are achieved, the characteristics of nonresponders should be investigated.

Attrition bias results when there is a systematic relevant difference between those retained and those lost to follow-up in cohort and experimental studies. Ideally, all baseline respondents should have equal probabilities of being retained in the study. In cohort studies of young injection drug users in Chicago, homeless, heavy-drug-using males are most likely to be lost to follow-up. The good news about retention bias is that it can be accurately evaluated, and study results can be adjusted appropriately. This is possible because relevant characteristics of nonresponders were collected at baseline. One evaluation method is to treat response/nonresponse as a dependent variable and examine relevant subject characteristics (e.g., gender, age, health status) as independent variables or predictors in regression models. Independent variables found to be significantly related to response/nonresponse can then be included as control variables in study models, thereby controlling their effects on the main relationship of interest (i.e., exposure and outcome). Similar to nonresponse bias, a retention rate less than 80% (less than 8 out of 10 baseline subjects are available in follow-up) is suggestive of bias and should be evaluated and reported.

STATISTICAL POWER ANALYSIS

We now know how to select subjects, but how many should we select? "It depends" is the short answer. The long answer involves conducting a power analysis. To understand the purpose of this analysis, let us first review Type I and Type II errors in hypothesis testing. These are illustrated in **Table 7–4**. Type I and Type II errors are the two types of mistakes we can make when deciding whether or not to reject a null hypothesis or accept a sample statistic as a valid estimate of a population parameter. Type I is the error we make when we REJECT a TRUE null hypothesis (incorrectly concluding we HAVE support for our alternative hypothesis when we actually should NOT reject the null hypothesis). This can be seen as a false-positive result. We assign a maximum probability for making this error, called alpha or α, usually as 0.05 or no greater than a 5% chance of making this mistake. Alternatively, we are 95% confident that our result is not due to chance and may be a real result.

Type II is the error we make when we do NOT reject a null hypothesis when the null hypothesis is really FALSE (incorrectly concluding we do NOT have support for our alternative hypothesis when we actually SHOULD reject the null hypothesis). This can be seen as a false negative. The maximum probability we assign to this error is usually 20%. This probability is represented by beta or β,

Table 7–4 Type I and Type II Errors

Reality	Decision	
	Reject null hypothesis (support for alternative hypothesis)	Fail to reject null hypothesis (no support for alternative hypothesis)
Null hypothesis is true (There really is no study result consistent with the alternative hypothesis.)	Type I error α 5%	Correct decision $(1 - \alpha)$ Significance level 95%
Null hypothesis is false (There really is a study result consistent with the alternative hypothesis.)	Correct decision $(1 - \beta)$ Power 80%	Type II error β 20%

and $(1 - \beta)$ is referred to the statistical power of our study. We want to have at least an 80% chance of rejecting a false null hypothesis. We want to have 80% power to detect real results in our study.

Statistical power depends largely on sample size. Generally, the larger the sample size, the higher the level of statistical power. Consider a confidence interval around the sample estimate of a population mean. The formula is:

$$\bar{X} \pm Z\left(\sigma/\sqrt{n}\right)$$

The confidence interval around the mean estimate includes the standard value of Z (representing the alpha of 0.05) and sample size n in the denominator. The larger the n, the smaller the interval will be. The smaller the interval, the more precise is the estimate. Knowing or assuming the sample mean and standard deviation σ and using the Z value with 95% confidence, we can solve for n using the above formula. Solving for n is a power analysis. The formulas we use for n depend on the study design and assumptions we must make about the sample population.

New and even seasoned researchers are encouraged to consult a statistician in the design stage of the study, particularly the power analysis. There are several power calculators available, many for free, on the Internet, so researchers can calculate the power needed for their particular study in terms of its specific design and assumptions. As a general illustration of what is required for a power analysis, we can discuss the necessary assumptions about sample populations and results for different study designs to determine the sample size needed for a study. The assumptions for different study designs are presented in **Table 7–5**. Typically, researchers strive to have at least 80% power (to avoid a Type II error) and at least 95% confidence (to avoid a Type I error). Minimally acceptable effect sizes vary by the nature of the study and clinical significance, and researchers can identify meaningful effect size estimates by reviewing relevant previous studies and/or conducting pilot tests. With these acceptable effect sizes as givens in the power analysis to solve for n, researchers must make a best estimate about ratios of group sizes and proportions with the exposure or the outcome. The more accurate the assumption, the more precise is the estimate of minimal sample size.

Again, statistical power is largely dependent on sample size, so the lazy researcher might just set out to include hundreds or thousands of subjects in the study without conducting a power analysis, assuming study funds will support large samples. Aside from a potential waste of money and time, this approach might be the incorrect one in two ways. First, with large samples, even very small

Table 7–5 Power Analysis Assumptions

Research question	Study design	Assumptions
What proportion of the population has the disorder?	Cross-sectional	1. Estimate of the proportion 2. Acceptable margin of error in the estimate (± ?) 3. Confidence level
Are cases more likely than controls to have been exposed to the potential cause?	Case-control	1. Ratio of controls to cases 2. Estimated proportion of controls who were exposed 3. Smallest odds ratio that would be a clinically meaningful result 4. Confidence level
Does the exposure affect the outcome?	Cohort	1. Ratio of unexposed to exposed 2. Estimated proportion of unexposed with outcome 3. Smallest risk ratio that would be clinically meaningful 4. Confidence level
Does the exposure affect the outcome?	Experiment	1. Ratio of experimental group to control group 2. Estimated proportion of controls with outcomes 3. Smallest risk ratio that would be clinically meaningful 4. Confidence level

and clinically insignificant measures of association will be found to be statistically significant. Depending on the nature of the study and the seriousness of the outcome, interpreting small effects as significant can be misleading and even harmful. Second, in experimental studies of exposures (e.g., drugs, procedures) that involve more than minimal risk, using a larger than necessary sample puts individuals at risk unnecessarily. Hence, a power analysis requires assumptions about statistical and clinical significance.

CONCLUSION

Obtaining a sample that sufficiently represents the target and sample populations requires a great deal of thought and anticipation. Sometimes, preliminary work such as a pilot test may be necessary to "get to know" the relevant characteristics of the target population. A sample that is much too small in terms of statistical power or significantly biased in relation to the target population is essentially useless. Samples that we end up with are rarely if ever exactly what we planned. Many times, we must adjust our analysis plan according to the limits of our sample. However, every reasonable effort should be made to define the appropriate target population, construct the best possible sampling frame, calculate the appropriate necessary sample size, correctly use the strongest possible sampling method, and effectively promote the study in order to recruit and retain the number and type of subjects needed to generate valid and meaningful results.

VOCABULARY

Alpha

Attrition bias

Beta

Convenience sample

Exclusionary criteria

External validity

Incentives

Inclusionary criteria

Internal validity

Modal instance
  sample

Nonprobability
  sampling

Nonresponse bias

Power analysis

Probability sampling

Purposive sample

Quota sample

Respondent-driven
  sampling

Recruitment

Retention

Sample

Sampling frame

Sampling method

Sample or study
  population

Screening

Selection bias

Simple random sample

Snowball sampling

Statistical power

Stratified random
  sample

Systematic random
  sample

Target or theoretical
  population

Type I error

Type II error

STUDY QUESTIONS AND EXERCISES

1. Describe an appropriate sampling frame for each of the following questions. Name one challenge to accessing each frame.
   a. What is the effect of banning menthol in cigarettes on smoking prevalence?
   b. What are the risk factors for the 2009 pandemic Influenza A (H1N1)?
   c. Is the new drug, carisoprodol (Soma), effective in treating sleep disorders?
   d. What factors are associated with injection drug users' sharing syringes?
2. Describe an appropriate sampling strategy for each of the research questions in problem 1. Name one limitation of each strategy.
3. Draft a recruitment letter for your study or for a hypothetical study. Be sure to include the necessary elements and make it as persuasive as possible.
4. Describe a potentially effective retention strategy for each of the following study samples.
   a. Homeless children in Brazil.
   b. Participants in a national trial testing the efficacy of a new drug for breast cancer.
   c. Substance use among high school students in Montreal.
   d. Adherence to medication among Mexican Americans with tuberculosis (TB).
5. What is the potential general probability (low, medium, high) of problematic nonresponse bias in each of the samples in problem 4? What procedures might minimize nonresponse bias for samples with a medium and high probability of such bias?
6. Draft the sampling protocol for your particular study idea. Include the following:
   a. Describe the target and study populations.
   b. Describe the sampling frame (if appropriate).
   c. Describe the sampling strategy.
   d. Describe the screening procedure (if appropriate).
   e. Describe the contact and recruitment procedures. (Include written materials as attachments.)
   f. Address the potential for nonresponse bias and how the bias may be minimized.
   g. Address the potential for attrition bias and how the bias may be minimized (if appropriate).

REFERENCES

Abdul-Quader, A. S., Heckathorn, D. D., Sabin, K., & Saidel, T. (2006, November). Implementation and analysis of respondent driven sampling: Lessons learned from the field. *Journal of Urban Health, 83*(6 Suppl), i1–5.

Boone L. E., & Kurtz, K. D. (2011). *Contemporary marketing 2011.* Mason, OH: South-Western.

Eyerman, J., Odom, D., Wu, S., & Butler, D. (2002). *Nonresponse in the 1999 NHSDA: Redesigning an ongoing national household survey, methodological issues* (No. SMA 03-3768). Rockville, MD: Substance Abuse and Mental Health Services Administration, Office of Applied Studies.

Heckathorn, D. D. (1997). Respondent-driven sampling: A new approach for studying hidden populations. *Social Problems, 44*(2), 174–199.

Heckathorn, D. D. (2011). Snowball versus respondent-driven sampling. *Sociological Methodology, 41*(1), 355–366.

Lee, E. S., & Forthofer, R. N. (2006). *Analyzing complex survey data* (2nd ed.). Thousand Oaks, CA: Sage Publications.

Magnani, R., Sabin, K., Saidel, T., & Heckathorn, D. (2005, May). Review of sampling hard-to-reach and hidden populations for HIV surveillance. *AIDS, 19*(Suppl 2), S67–72.

Substance Abuse and Mental Health Services Administration. (2010). *Results from the 2009 national survey on drug use and health: Volume 1. Summary of national findings* (No. SMA 10-4586). Rockville, MD: Substance Abuse and Mental Health Services Administration, Office of Applied Studies.

United States Census Bureau. (2002). Summary population and housing characteristics. *2000 census of population and housing* (No. PH-1-1). Washington, DC: United States Government Printing Office.

CHAPTER 8

Measuring Concepts

LEARNING OBJECTIVES

By the end of this chapter the reader will be able to:

- Explain the processes of measuring concepts and collecting data.
- Distinguish between different types of measurement techniques.
- Measure concepts and collect data using different data collection techniques.

CHAPTER OUTLINE

Conceptualization, operationalization—what is that?

INTRODUCTION

Measuring data or designing instruments to collect data is an essential step in the research process. The instrument could be a survey, questionnaire, diagnosis, or lab test, depending on the study purpose. Designing an instrument involves conceptualization, construction, pretesting, and administration. The steps in this process often overlap.

Conceptualization usually refers to defining the target population and what is being measured. In the interest of validity and reliability, particular care should be taken to define as precisely as possible what variables are being measured and how. Operationalization is the process of translating concepts into actual measurements. The process takes the research concepts from the minds of researchers to observable and replicable measures. Successful operationalization is conducted with a focus on validity (measuring what is intended) and reliability (consistency across subjects and measurement points). The intended result of the operationalization process is measurement that is observable and presented in a detailed, thorough, and specific way that can be repeated or replicated by other researchers (Burns & Grove, 2005).

For example, research studies have demonstrated that fruit and vegetable intake are beneficial for an individual's health. This is an interesting area of research, so a research scientist proposes to test the hypothesis, "Eating fruits and vegetables provides adequate fiber intake that can help lower blood cholesterol levels among males." This is a good topic for research; however it does need some clarification and strengthening (i.e., it needs operationalization). The researcher needs to define and make measurable what exactly is "adequate" or beneficial intake of fruits and vegetables. How much? How many? What type? How often? With a strong, precise definition of "adequate" intake, the researcher must then determine the best possible and practical ways to measure intake. Should food be weighed or measured? Should servings at different meals be counted separately? Are self-reports valid? Are food diaries reliable? Is a prescribed diet feasible? All important issues and options should be explored.

As a further introduction to methods of measurement and data collection, the concept of measurement level should be reviewed. Stanly Stevens articulated the four-level system of measurement in 1946. These levels range from lower to higher in the order of categorical (nominal and dichotomous), ordinal, and continuous (interval and ratio). They rank from lowest to highest in terms of complexity, precision, and the analytic options they facilitate. Categorical or nominal scales are the simplest and lowest scale of measurement. This scale of measurement is used when data can be organized only in categories or classes. For example, gender and eye color are measured as categories. The categories cannot be ordered from lowest to highest or highest to lowest in any meaningful way. It involves a simple count of frequency of the cases in various categories. Ordinal scales are used when measurement categories can be ranked or ordered. Classes of categories such as low, medium, or high heart rate or intensity of agreement to the importance of adequate fruit intake (not at all important to very important) are examples of ordinal measures. The categories do not have inherently meaningful numeric values and the intervals between them are unequal. From ordinal variables, the researcher can understand the order of preference, but nothing about how much more one choice is preferred to another. Statistics such as median, quartile, and percentile can be calculated with ordinal variables (Burns & Grove, 2005; Monsen & Van Horn, 2008).

Interval scales have numerically equal distance between categories of the scale. Interval scales help indicate the magnitude of the difference. Temperature measured in degrees Celsius is an example of an interval scale. The differences between 2 and 3 degrees and between 42 and 43 degrees are the same—1 degree. Most of the statistical methods of analysis require interval variables. Ratio scales are the highest level of measurement. This level has all the properties of the previous three levels (characteristics, rank order, and equal distance between intervals) and in addition, it has a fixed origin or zero point. Ratio scales permit the researcher to compare both the differences in and also the relative magnitude of scores. With ratio scales, one can say that subject A weighs twice as much as subject B. These four levels of measurement play an important role in research, as each level of measurement is associated with the type of statistical analyses that can be conducted on that particular variable (Burns & Grove, 2005; Monsen & Van Horn, 2008).

Once the variables and appropriate levels of measurement have been determined and operational definitions have been assigned, the process of instrument construction can begin. Construction refers to writing questions for surveys or questionnaires, stipulating criteria for biological measurement, calibrating instrumentation, and testing the reliability, validity, objectivity, and usability of the tool. Reliability, validity, objectivity, and usability can be determined from previous studies or tested in pilot or pretests of the instrumentation.

The process of collecting information from selected subjects is called data collection. The procedure for collecting data varies according to the research design and the objective of the research project. Data can be collected by observing, testing, measuring, or asking questions. Before initiating data collection, specific procedures should be determined and defined. First, a correct data collection method and tool should be selected. The researcher should make sure, as thoroughly as possible, that the data collection tool is reliable and standardized. Second, the complete practical steps to collect the data should be specified in detail and recorded in the study. These steps include information about where specifically the data will be collected (measurement site), who will collect it, precise collection procedures, and exit instructions (Burns & Grove, 2005).

Some important points to consider when planning data collection procedures are (1) credibility—assuring the data collected is relevant and measures important information; (2) validity—actually measuring what the instrument is intended to measure; and (3) reliability—producing consistent measures with the same tool in repeated tests.

SURVEY DATA COLLECTION

The survey is a commonly used technique for collecting data. Surveys are an efficient and often effective vehicle for measuring perceptions, opinions, and ideas. When it comes to measuring behavior, surveys are often less accurate, as what people say may be different from what they actually do. Giving false answers about behavior or any other concept is called prevarication bias. Sensitive and illegal behaviors are subject to this type of bias and should be verified if possible (e.g., drug tests, court records). In any event, survey research has been used to measure concepts such as perceptions of health, self-efficacy of limiting fat intake, and perceived quality of Internet-based distance learning.

Surveys can be used for description, explanation, and exploration. A researcher might select a survey technique for the purpose of gathering descriptive data about some population, or data about some particular characteristics of the population. On the other hand, some other studies, in addition to description, will try to make some explanatory assertions of the population. Surveys can also be used as a "search device" when you are working with a particularly new research topic about which little is known. This is called an exploratory survey. Many researchers use more than one such objective in their studies. Once the purpose of the survey is finalized, survey design begins. There are two basic survey designs: cross-sectional and longitudinal surveys (Babbie, 1990).

In cross-sectional surveys, data are collected at one point in time. Cross-sectional surveys can be used for description purposes as well as to determine the relationship between variables at the time of the study. Longitudinal surveys collect data at different points in time (e.g., baseline and follow-up), and changes in behaviors or opinions or other factors are measured. The most common longitudinal designs are trend studies and cohort studies. In trend studies, the general population is sampled at different points in time. Different individuals are sampled for each survey; however, each sample should represent the same population and hence provide the trend data for that particular population. Cohort studies focus on the same specific population each time the data are collected. The same individuals are surveyed at baseline and subsequent follow-up measures.

Surveys can be either structured or semi-structured. Structured surveys have a predetermined range of responses that the respondent can select. This structure ensures that all the subjects are given the exact same question and choices of answers. Semi-structured questionnaires include questions with response options, but leave some or most of the questions open-ended so that respondents can answer in their own words, reflecting their own conceptualizations of their responses (Babbie, 1990; Malhotra, 2006). Below are examples of both types of questions.

Example of a structured question:
How confident are you that you will exercise when your exercise partner decides not to exercise that day?

Not at all confident	Somewhat confident	Moderately confident	Very confident	Completely confident

Example of a semi-structured question:
Based on your lifestyle intervention classes, what are the two major benefits of participating in regular physical activity? (1) _____
(2)_____

Developing a survey instrument can be a research study in itself. When possible, the researcher starts with questions used successfully by prior studies. In some or perhaps most cases, however, new questions measuring new concepts must be created. With new questions and/or possibly new target populations, it is essential to pretest the tool with a small but fairly representative group of subjects. Feedback from this pretesting facilitates appropriate revisions. Studies that develop new surveys or scales on a particular topic must establish the validity and reliability of the tool themselves.

Survey Construction

Three important aspects of survey instruments are (1) types of questions, (2) question wording, and (3) question placement. Typically, surveys are thought to just include a series of questions. However, most, if not all, surveys include a series of statements as well. The use of both questions and statements provides more flexibility in the design of the questionnaire. Some of the choices of the types of questions are structure (closed- or open-ended), level of measurement (dichotomous, categorical, ordinal, continuous), and purpose (filter/contingency, transition).

Closed-ended questions are more popular in survey research because they provide uniformity of responses and are easily processed for data analysis. Two necessary requirements for closed-ended questions are that (1) response categories should be exhaustive (all possible responses should be included), and (2) they should be mutually exclusive (there should be no overlap between categories). For example, a survey question about personal income should include choices at the low and high end of the possible income range (e.g., less than $10,000 per year; more than $150,000 per year) to be truly exhaustive. Categorical measures often include an "Other" response option in order to be exhaustive. Again for the example of income, there should be no overlap in values for category choices (e.g., not $20,000–$30,000; then $30,000–$40,000) for the choices to be mutually exclusive. In this example, an individual who earns exactly $30,000 per year could choose either the first or the second of these categories. These types of mistakes threaten the validity of responses (Malhotra, 2006).

Dichotomous questions have two possible responses. Examples of dichotomous choices are male/female, yes/no, and true/false. Categorical questions have nonnumerical responses that cannot be ordered. Some of the examples of this type of question are occupation, race/ethnicity, and residence. For example:

Specify your race:

_____ American Indian or Alaska Native
_____ Asian
_____ Black or African American
_____ Native Hawaiian or Other Pacific Islander
_____ White
_____ Other

Ordinal questions also provide categorical response options; however, the nonnumeric responses can be ordered in a meaningful way. Responses based on Likert scales are an excellent example of ordinal questions. Likert scale responses are ratings based on a scale that has been assigned to the response. These questions usually range from strongly agree to strongly disagree. Questions that have responses with meaningful numeric values are classified as continuous questions.

These can be either interval or ratio. Examples of continuous measures include blood pressure, income, and weight. These types of measures are often best collected by research staff in that self-reports have highly questionable validity. When a survey is the only possible measurement mechanism, concepts should be carefully defined and measurement procedures may need to be described for subjects.

Sometimes survey questions serve a practical function intended to assist in the successful progress through the instrument. In addition to measuring concepts, these questions are intended to assist the understanding of the respondent, and, consequently, the validity of the measure. One major example of functional questions is filter or contingency questions. Responses to a filter question will determine if a follow-up question is appropriate or if it would make more sense to the respondent to skip to the next topic or the next groups of questions. For example:

Have you ever been convicted of a felony?
_____Yes _____No
Follow-up question:
If yes, how many times? _____once; _____2 to 5 times;
_____6 to 10 times; _____more than 10 times

Once the type of question has been determined, it is important to check the content and the wording of the question. Make sure that the question is measuring what it is supposed to measure. If it "appears" to measure the correct concept, then it is said to have good "face" validity. On the face of it, it appears to be appropriate. This is a minimal requirement for validity. (Tests for measurement validity and reliability are discussed later.) Generally, concepts should be defined so that the respondent perceives the concept as the researcher intended. The level of language used should be appropriate for the audience. Is it reasonable to expect that the subjects would understand certain terms such as cholesterol or tumor? If not, they should be defined clearly. When in doubt, define it. If the survey is self-administered, the lowest appropriate reading level (e.g., sixth grade level) should be used. (There are online programs available to test reading levels.) Construct clear and briefly worded questions and avoid using wording that suggests the opinions of the researcher. Finally, every effort should be made to avoid wording that might be threatening to the respondent. Types of terms and wordings to be avoided include:

1. Pejorative terms (i.e., racial slurs)
2. Judgments (i.e., expressions of opinion)
3. Insensitive wording about sensitive topics (e.g., how wealthy are you?)

The format of a questionnaire is as important as the wording and construction of the questionnaire. The text in the questionnaire should be uncluttered, and white space should be maximized. Point size should be as large as required for ease of reading. Placement of questions (ordering of questions) is also an important part of survey construction. There should be logic in ordering the questions. Questions at the start of the survey should be easy to answer, interesting, and nonthreatening for the subjects. Sensitive questions should be embedded in the middle, and demographic questions should be at the end of the survey. Questions vital to the purpose of the study (i.e., dimensions of the exposure) should not be placed at the end of the survey because some proportion of subjects will not complete the survey. A clear numbering system for questions helps respondents navigate correctly through all the questions.

Questions should be grouped by themes or topics. When changing themes or topics, transition statements help the subjects change gears in their thinking, as in this example: "Now, we'd like to ask a few questions about your consumption of energy drinks. Energy drinks include . . ." As demonstrated in this example, the change of topic is clear, and the transition provides an opportunity to define terms for maximizing validity. It is also helpful to leave some white space (visual distinction) between different topics. Whenever possible, questions with the same response format should be grouped together. For example, all multiple response questions together, all Likert scales together, and so on.

The survey should be as short, simple, and nonthreatening as possible. Researchers should put themselves in the place of the respondent and ask themselves: "Would you complete this survey?" "Would you skip this question?" "Would this question offend you?" If the survey respondents are different from researchers on relevant characteristics (e.g., age, cognitive ability), then the survey should be pretested with a small group of subjects with these characteristics. In addition, the interviewer should explore issues of question formatting, wording, and placement in the pretest. Again, the most important tone of the survey and study is "respect." Thank the respondents before and after the survey for taking the time to respond. It should be made clear that their time and effort are important and greatly appreciated (Malhotra, 2006; Babbie, 1990).

Advantages of Survey Research

Written surveys are relatively inexpensive and a large amount of data from a large number of people can be collected in a relatively short period of time. Another advantage is that there is lower variability in data collection, as every individual is exposed to a similar stimulus. Structured surveys take longer to develop, but are easier to administer and analyze. When working with a large sample size, structured surveys are more efficient compared to semi-structured surveys or other methods. On the other hand, the semi-structured surveys are easier to develop and provide very rich data and concepts not anticipated by the researcher.

Disadvantages of Survey Research

One of the major concerns with survey research is response rate. In ideal conditions for results to be representative of the population, the response rate should be 100%—every respondent participates. However, studies have indicated that response rates are usually lower than 100%. A rate of 80% or higher is generally considered acceptable. A study with a lower rate should be examined for response bias. Known characteristics of responders and nonresponders should be compared to see if there are any systematic differences that might influence the results. Similarly, it is reasonable to expect that some respondents will not complete the entire survey for a variety of reasons. Respondents who complete less than 80% of the survey should be compared to those who complete 80% or more to see if there are systematic differences. If bias is suggested, then the incomplete survey should be dropped from the data set, and the response rate adjusted accordingly (Babbie, 1990).

VALIDITY AND RELIABILITY OF MEASURES

Measurement bias and error are distinct threats to the value of study results. What a loss to spend the time, energy, and money to collect data that is biased. Because of this threat, time and attention should be devoted to measurement validity and reliability in the planning and piloting stages of the study. Validity refers to the ability of the instrument to measure what it is intended to measure. Picture a target with a bull's eye. Validity is achieved when the shooter hits the bull's eye. How well does a measure represent the "truth" or true concept? Reliability is the ability of the tool to yield consistent findings. Back to the target analogy, reliability is achieved to the extent that the shooter hits the same area of the target. Ideally, the shooter will hit the bull's eye repeatedly and achieve validity and reliability (Burns & Grove, 2005).

Criteria for measurement validity and reliability and ways to evaluate them are:

1. *Predictive validity*—ability of the measure to predict something it should, theoretically, be able to predict (e.g., a measure of depression should predict suicide ideation)
2. *Concurrent validity*—ability of the measure to distinguish between groups that it theoretically should be able to distinguish between (e.g., a measure of depression should distinguish depressed persons from anxious persons)
3. *Convergent validity*—degree to which the measure is similar to other measures it theoretically should be similar to (e.g., a measure of depression should be able to identify depressed persons as well as the Diagnostic and Statistical Manual of Mental Disorders [*DSM-IV*] criteria diagnoses depressed persons)
4. *Discriminant validity*—degree to which the measure is dissimilar to other measures to which it theoretically should not be similar to (e.g., a measure of depression should be substantively different from a measure of anxiety)
5. *Inter-rater reliability*—degree to which different raters give consistent estimates of the same phenomena (e.g., two trained interviewers should be able to identify the same subject as being depressed)
6. *Test-retest reliability*—degree to which a measure performs consistently from one time to another (e.g., the same instrument should identify the same subject as being depressed over two administrations separated by a short period of time)
7. *Parallel-forms reliability*—degree to which similar measures of the same construct provide consistent results (e.g., two similar measures of depression—perhaps with different wording or response options—should both identify depressed subjects)
8. *Internal consistency*—degree to which responses are consistent across items representing components of an overall construct (e.g., components of the measure of depression such as changes in appetite and lack of interest in previous activities should elicit consistent responses)

Ideally, results of the new measure can be compared to those of some accepted gold-standard measure with known reliability and validity. If no such measure is available, and perhaps even if it is, researchers should test measures using multiple criteria and testing methods before using the instrument in main study.

Reliability can be measured quantitatively with Cronbach's alpha or reliability coefficient. Generally, the measure represents how often ratings between interviewers or across measurement periods match. A measure that is completely reliable will have a coefficient of 1.0 (ratings always agree), and one that is totally unreliable will have a coefficient of 0.0 (ratings never agree). Typically, a coefficient of 0.75 or higher (75% agreement) is considered acceptable.

Survey research is subject to bias resulting from measurement error. Unreliable and invalid survey measures are a real threat in survey designs. The environment in which the survey is conducted, the way the questions are drafted and placed, and the state of the respondent can all influence the measurement. When possible, survey items tested in other studies should be adopted. When this is not possible, preliminary work on questions is worth the time and effort to help maximize validity. The survey can be administered to a pilot group, after which a focus group is created with respondents to discuss the items in detail. What did the respondents think a question meant to ask about? How do the respondents define key terms? Was the wording confusing in any way? Were all relevant response options included? Additionally, cognitive tests can be implemented to explore in detail the perceived meaning and interpretation of survey questions. These are relevant strategies in addition to comparing survey items to a gold-standard measure (biological tests, medical records, etc.).

SCALES

Scales are often used for measuring complex phenomena. Guttman scales combine multiple components representing all relevant aspects of the concept of interest. For example, a scale measuring depression would combine, perhaps in an additive fashion, components of feeling sad or blue, change in sleep patterns, change in appetite, lack of interest in activities, suicide ideation, and so on. For itemized rating scales, a brief description or number is assigned to each response category. Individual responses are then combined mathematically to form a more complex scale.

The term *scale* is also used to describe the level of measurement of response choices in survey items. Examples are Likert scales, rating scales, and semantic differential scales.

Likert Scales

Likert scales consist of a number of declarative statements with a value assigned to each statement. The scale usually ranges between "strongly agree" and "strongly

Table 8–1 Example of a Likert Scale

	Almost always	Often	Sometimes	Seldom	Never
Do you have any say in buying foods for your family?	☐	☐	☐	☐	☐
Do you decide what you eat at school?	☐	☐	☐	☐	☐
Do you have any say in how food is prepared at home?	☐	☐	☐	☐	☐

disagree." Respondents indicate their degree of agreement by checking one of the five responses: "strongly disagree," "disagree," "neither agree nor disagree," "agree," and "strongly agree." The original and most common format of the Likert scale has five response categories with a value of 1 assigned to the most negative response and a value of 5 assigned to the most positive response. The middle category typically represents a neutral response. Likert data is typically treated as an interval scale. Researchers may wish respondents to choose a response that is not neutral. In this case, they may use a four- or six-response category option. This type of scale (where the neutral response is omitted) is known as a forced-choice version. Likert scale instruments usually include 10 to 20 items, each designed to measure the concept of interest. Researchers should mix positive and negative items in the group for the scale to assure that respondents are paying attention to the content of the questions and not simply choosing the same response for every item. When analyzing Likert data, it is important to follow a consistent scoring procedure (Babbie, 1990; Burns & Grove, 2005; Malhotra, 2006). **Table 8–1** shows items that could be included in a Likert scale.

Rating Scales

Rating scales are the crudest form of scaling techniques. An ordered series of category choices are listed on a numeric continuum. For example, respondents may be asked to rate items in order of priority or interest. Rating scales provide numerical data with specific or anchored endpoints. Items for a rating scale can be presented in text or graphic form (Burns & Grove, 2005). **Figure 8–1** shows two examples of rating scales (text and graphic).

Student evaluation of the presentation skills: Circle the appropriate number, using the following key: 5 = Excellent, 4 = Above Average, 3 = Average, 2 = Below Average, 1 = Poor.	Student evaluation of the teaching skills: Rate the presenter by placing an X anywhere along each line.
1. Covered the material in detail 1 2 3 4 5	1. Covers the material in detail Always | Frequently | Occasionally | Seldom | Never
2. Presented the material clearly 1 2 3 4 5	2. Presented the material clearly Always | Frequently | Occasionally | Seldom | Never
3. Involved the audience 1 2 3 4 5	3. Involved the audience Always | Frequently | Occasionally | Seldom | Never

FIGURE 8–1 Text and Graphic Examples of Rating Scales

Semantic Differential Scales

Semantic differential scales present response options on a visual continuum with two defined endpoints and simple numbers in between. Typically, there is a 7-point scale between the two endpoints, and respondents are asked to select the number on the scale that best expresses their belief or opinion. This scale is used to measure attitudes or beliefs of respondents. Values from 1 to 7 are assigned to each space on the scale, with 1 being the most negative response and 7 being the most positive response. The placement of the negative responses to the left or right of the scale on the survey tool should be varied to avoid global or thoughtless responses. In the field of health research, the traditional semantic differential scale has been modified and called the semantic differential for health (Jenkins, 1966; Osgood, Suci, & Tannenbaum 1957). These health-based semantic scales have been used to estimate health-relevant perceptions. Factor analysis is used to evaluate the validity of this scale and distinguish the themes (Burns & Grove, 2005; Monsen & Van Horn, 2008). **Figure 8–2** shows an example of a health-based semantic differential scale (e.g., beliefs about cancer).

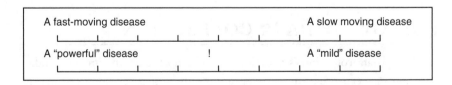

FIGURE 8–2 Example of a Health-Based Semantic Differential Scale: Beliefs About Cancer

CLINICAL DATA COLLECTION

Clinical data collection focuses on a data collection schedule (timing of measurement) and related forms (instruments, type of measurement) for data collection. These two steps will determine the amount and quantity of data that will be gathered. The study protocol should state clearly what instruments or forms should be used at which measurement time point.

Form development is usually initiated by reviewing the literature for instruments used in similar studies. Form development requires background research and pilot testing. In pilot testing, the use of real patients as a test sample provides good estimates for the validity of the tool as well as an estimate of data collection times. Based on the results of the pilot testing, changes should be incorporated in the tool.

Once the data collection starts, it is important that all the required initial data for the subjects be collected during the initial visit. This should include a checklist (screener) with inclusion and exclusion criteria to determine subject eligibility. Once the patients are enrolled in the study, baseline data should be collected. If the study is a randomized controlled trial, patients should be randomized into treatment or control groups following their baseline evaluation. Required follow-up visits should be scheduled after this initial visit. The purpose and procedures of each visit should be clearly communicated to the patient. During the follow-up visits, data on treatment compliance and any side effects should be collected (Weinstein & Deyo, 2000).

For example, a study is being conducted to evaluate the effect of a lifestyle intervention on improving patients' blood glucose and lipid profiles. The lifestyle intervention focuses on healthy eating and regular (5 days a week) physical activity. The intervention will last 6 months and will include nutrition lessons, physical activity workshops, and cooking classes. Pre- and postintervention data will be collected to evaluate the efficacy of the intervention on improving blood glucose and lipid profiles. **Table 8–2** shows an abbreviated data collection form.

FOLLOW-UP DATA COLLECTION

Follow-up data collection is a vital aspect of cohort and experimental studies. Attrition bias can occur and weaken an already expensive and time-intensive study when more than 20% of the baseline group is lost before the final follow-up data are collected. Because of the strength of these study designs in their ability to

Table 8–2 Example of an Abbreviated Data Collection Form

	Date (pre-data)	Date (mid-point data, 3 months)	Date (post-data, 6 months)
Demographics: Gender Age (years) Ethnicity	X		X
Labs: Blood glucose (mg/dL) Total cholesterol (mg/dL) HDL (mg/dL) LDL (mg/dL) Triglycerides (mg/dL)	X	X	X
Anthropometrics: Height (inches) Weight (pounds) Body mass index Waist circumference (inches)	X		X

X = denotes data collection times

demonstrate causality and the time and money already invested, every reasonable and affordable effort should be made to maintain and follow-up subjects in the study. Follow-up can be either active or passive.

Active Follow-Up

During active follow-up, the investigator is the point of contact with the cohort. He or she directly contacts cohort members, updates contact information, and obtains data that may show incidence of disease or changes in risk factors or biological markers. Follow-up data collection techniques usually involve mailed questionnaires, phone calls, Internet contacts, or written invitations to return to the site for in-person data collection. This follow-up method demands a great deal of financial and staff resources (Friis & Sellers, 2009).

Passive Follow-Up

During passive follow-up, the investigator does not contact cohort members directly. This type of follow-up is possible when an external database management team is used to maintain and collect data on outcomes of interest. Such data management is possible for diseases or conditions for which federal and state governments mandate reporting. The cancer registry is an example of this type of data surveillance. It is possible for investigators to link records from these databases to data collected directly from the study cohort (Friis & Sellers, 2009).

SECONDARY SOURCES

Secondary data or existing data have been collected by other investigators and are publically available for others to analyze. In secondary data analysis, the people involved in data analyses are usually not involved in actual data collection or designing the methodology for data collection. For example, a researcher develops a research question that can be addressed through analysis of data available from the National Health and Nutrition Examination Survey (NHANES), a data set that is collected every 4 years by the National Center for Health Statistics (NCHS, a part of the Centers for Disease Control and Prevention). In this example, the researcher intending to analyze this data set did not participate in designing this study or in the process of data collection. Ideally, data documentation is available with the public data set. The best documentation would include the overall study protocol (explaining every step of the study), data collection procedures, instruments, and details about data processing, including entry, recodes, variable construction, treatment of missing data, and variable frequencies. Such documentation should allow the researcher to analyze and interpret the data in the context of understanding what the data measures really mean, as if she was part of the study design and data collection stages of the study (Bibb, 2007; Boslaugh, 2007).

Advantages and Disadvantages of Secondary Data Analysis

Most researchers in epidemiology work with both primary and secondary data. One of the major advantages of working with secondary data analysis is cost savings. The data has already been collected by someone, so the researcher does not have to set aside money for data collection. Sometimes the researcher does have to pay for access to secondary data sets; however, such costs are minimal compared to the considerable costs involved in collecting primary data. Conserving time is another advantage of using secondary data. As the data is already collected, cleaned, and stored in an electronic format, the researcher is free to focus on data analyses.

Another added advantage of the secondary databases is the breadth of data that is available in these data sets. An independent researcher might not have enough resources to collect a representative sample of all U.S. adults. Moreover, many of these studies are repeated at a set interval of time, providing an opportunity to analyze data longitudinally. Many of these data sets use complex sampling designs and collect data on a large sample size, thus increasing the generalizability of results. In addition, utilized data collection tools are often highly valid and reliable, thus increasing the accuracy of the data. Using these well designed databases, the researcher can draw population-based estimates of health conditions and behaviors. Due to these advantages, the use of secondary data sets for master's level research projects results in high quality with little cost. However, high-quality results are only possible when conducting high-quality analyses (Bibb, 2007; Boslaugh, 2007).

The main disadvantage of secondary databases is that they are not necessarily designed to answer a secondary researcher's specific research questions. Important data may not have been collected. If collected, it may not have been coded or categorized appropriately relative to the research question, and certain confidential information might not be available to the secondary researcher. Hence, the research question will likely need to be revised relative to the data that exist in these databases. Secondly, as the researcher is not a part of the study design or data collection tool, she may not have a good understanding of exactly how the study was conducted. This understanding can only be as good as the available documentation for the data (Bibb, 2007; Boslaugh, 2007; Schneeweiss, 2007).

There are several secondary databases that are available to the researcher at no cost. An excellent listing of all public health secondary databases is presented and discussed in Sarah Boslaugh's *Secondary Data Sources for Public Health: A Practical Guide* (2007). With so many governmental and private databases available for researchers, it makes the selection process of databases complicated. Some of the common health-related databases are listed in **Table 8–3**. The majority of these can be located on the National Center for Health Statistics (NCHS) and U.S. Department of Health and Human Services (DHHS) websites (see Table 8–3) (Centers for Disease Control and Prevention [CDC], 2012). Epidemiological data are accessible from a variety of sources ranging from vital statistics to reports of absenteeism from work. Some examples of epidemiological databases are disease registries, mortality statistics, health insurance data, hospital patient data, school health program data, labor statistics, and so on. Data from these sources can be used for descriptive as well as analytical studies. Investigators analyzing secondary data should be educated about the details of the data collection procedures (e.g., sampling frames and techniques, measures, data processing) so that potential biases can be addressed. In addition, secondary data analysis should not replicate exactly what has been analyzed previously, and researchers should always cite the original source of the data as well as relevant previous studies using the data (Bibb, 2007; Boslaugh, 2007).

Table 8–3 List of Selected Publically Available Databases

Database	Source	Brief description
National Health and Nutrition Examination Survey (NHANES)	CDC and NCHS, http://www.cdc.gov/nchs/nhanes.htm	NHANES is designed to assess the health and nutritional status of adults and children in the United States. The survey is unique in that it combines interviews and physical examinations. It began in early 1960s and has been conducted since then as a series of surveys. In 1999, the survey became a continuous program with focus on a variety of health and nutrition measurements to meet emerging needs. The survey examines a nationally representative sample of about 5,000 persons each year. The NHANES interview includes demographic, socioeconomic, dietary, and health-related questions. The examination component consists of medical, dental, and physiological measurements, as well as laboratory tests administered by highly trained medical personnel.
National Hospital Care Survey	CDC and NCHS, http://www.cdc.gov/nchs/nhcs.htm	The NHCS is designed to answer key questions of interest to healthcare policy makers, public health professionals, and researchers. Some of these factors include the use of healthcare resources, the quality of health care including safety, and disparities in healthcare services provided to population subgroups in the United States. These surveys use a combination of design features that make them unique. The surveys are nationally representative, provider-based, and cover a broad spectrum of healthcare settings.
National Ambulatory Medical Care Survey (NAMCS)	CDC and NCHS, http://www.cdc.gov/nchs/ahcd.htm	The NAMCS is designed to meet the need for objective, reliable information about the provision and use of ambulatory medical care services in the United States. Findings are based on a sample of visits to non-federally employed, office-based physicians who are primarily engaged in direct patient care.
National Hospital Ambulatory Medical Care Survey (NHAMCS)	CDC and NCHS, http://www.cdc.gov/nchs/ahcd.htm	The NHAMCS is designed to collect data on the utilization and provision of ambulatory care services in hospital emergency and outpatient departments. Findings are based on a national sample of visits to the emergency departments and outpatient departments of noninstitutional general and short-stay hospitals.
National Hospital Discharge Survey (NHDS)	CDC and NCHS, http://www.cdc.gov/nchs/nhds.htm	The NHDS is designed to meet the need for nationally representative information on inpatients discharged from nonfederal short-stay hospitals in the United States. In 2007, approximately 366,000 inpatient records were obtained from 422 hospitals. Beginning in 2008 the sample was reduced to 239 hospitals. The most recent survey was conducted in 2010.

(continued)

Table 8–3 List of Selected Publically Available Databases *(Cont'd)*

Database	Source	Brief description
National Survey of Ambulatory Surgery (NSAS)	CDC and NCHS, http://www.cdc.gov/nchs/nsas.htm	The NSAS is the only nationally representative sample of ambulatory surgery visits. In 2006, data was collected from hospital-based and freestanding ambulatory surgery facilities for the first time in 10 years.
National Health Interview Survey (NHIS)	CDC and NCHS, DHHS, http://www.cdc.gov/nchs/nhis.htm	The main objective of the NHIS is to monitor the health of the U.S. population through the collection and analysis of data on a broad range of health topics. This is a cross-sectional household interview survey. Sampling and interviewing are continuous throughout each year. The sampling plan follows a multistage area probability design that permits the representative sampling of households and noninstitutional group quarters. The sampling plan is redesigned after every decennial census.
National Health Interview Survey on Disability (NHIS-D)	http://www.cdc.gov/nchs/nhis/nhis_disability.htm	NHIS-D's objective is to develop a series of questionnaires that would provide a useful set of measures while maintaining a balance between the social, administrative, and medical considerations involved in disability measurement. It is designed to collect data that can be used to understand disability, to develop public health policy, to produce simple prevalence estimates of selected health conditions, and to provide descriptive baseline statistics on the effects of disabilities.
Joint Canada/United States Survey of Health (JCUSH)	http://www.cdc.gov/nchs/nhis/jcush.htm	The JCUSH was a research study conducted jointly by the National Center for Health Statistics and Statistics Canada. Data collection began in November 2002 and ended in March 2003. The JCUSH was a one-time, random telephone survey in both countries. Approximately 3,500 Canadian and 5,200 U.S. residents participated in the study.
National Immunization Survey (NIS)	National Center for Immunizations and Respiratory Diseases (NCIRD), NCHS, CDC, http://www.cdc.gov/nchs/nis.htm	The NIS is sponsored by the NCIRD and conducted jointly by NCIRD and the NCHS and CDC. The NIS is a list-assisted random-digit-dialing telephone survey followed by a mailed survey to children's immunization providers that began data collection in April 1994 to monitor childhood immunization coverage. Children between the ages of 19 and 35 months living in the United States at the time of the interview were included.
Longitudinal Studies of Aging (LSOA)	NCHS and National Institute on Aging (NIA), http://www.cdc.gov/nchs/lsoa.htm	LSOA is a multicohort study of persons 70 years of age and older designed primarily to measure changes in the health, functional status, living arrangements, and health services utilization of two cohorts of Americans as they move into and through the oldest ages.

(continued)

Table 8–3 List of Selected Publically Available Databases *(Cont'd)*

Database	Source	Brief description
State and Local Area Integrated Telephone Survey (SLAITS)	CDC and NCHS, http://www.cdc.gov/nchs/slaits.htm	SLAITS collects healthcare data at state and local levels. This data supplements current national data collection strategies by providing in-depth state and local area data.
		SLAITS provides a mechanism to collect data quickly on a broad range of topics at the national, state, and local levels. A partial list of examples of research areas includes health insurance coverage, access to care, perceived health status, utilization of services, and measurement of child well-being.
National Vital Statistics System (NVSS)	CDC and NCHS, http://www.cdc.gov/nchs/nvss.htm	In the United States, legal authority for the registration of these events resides individually within the 50 States, 2 cities (Washington, DC, and New York City), and 5 territories (Puerto Rico, the U.S. Virgin Islands, Guam, American Samoa, and the Commonwealth of the Northern Mariana Islands). These jurisdictions are responsible for maintaining registries of vital events and for issuing copies of birth, marriage, divorce, and death certificates.
Birth Data	http://www.cdc.gov/nchs/births.htm	In the United States, state laws require birth certificates to be completed for all births, and federal law mandates national collection and publication of births and other vital statistics data.
Mortality Data	http://www.cdc.gov/nchs/deaths.htm	Mortality data from the NVSS are an important source of demographic, geographic, and cause-of-death information. This is one of the few sources of health-related data that are comparable for small geographic areas and are available for a long time period in the United States. The data are also used to present the characteristics of those dying in the United States, to determine life expectancy, and to compare mortality trends with other countries.
Fetal Death Data	http://www.cdc.gov/nchs/fetal_death.htm#Methods	Fetal death data is published annually by the NCHS in reports and as individual-record data files. In the United States, state laws require the reporting of fetal deaths and federal law mandates national collection and publication of fetal death data.
Linked Birth and Infant Death Data	http://www.cdc.gov/nchs/linked.htm	The linked birth and infant death data set is a valuable tool for monitoring and exploring the complex interrelationships between infant death and risk factors present at birth. The linked files include information from the birth certificate such as age, race, Hispanic origin of the parents, birth weight, period of gestation, plurality, prenatal care usage, maternal

(continued)

Table 8–3 List of Selected Publically Available Databases *(Cont'd)*

Database	Source	Brief description
		education, live birth order, marital status, and maternal smoking, linked to information from the death certificate such as age at death and underlying and multiple causes of death.
National Mortality Followback Survey	http://www.cdc.gov/nchs/nvss/nmfs.htm	The Mortality Followback Survey began in the 1960s and uses a sample of U.S. residents who die in a given year to supplement the death certificate with information from the next of kin or another person familiar with the decedent's life history. This information, sometimes enhanced by administrative records, provides a unique opportunity to study the etiology of disease, demographic trends in mortality, and other health issues. This survey has evolved over time. In 1961: data on hospital and institutional care in the last year of life was collected; 1962–1963: an extensive analysis of socioeconomic differentials in mortality was collected; 1964–1965: expenditures for health care during the last year of life, sources of payment, and health insurance coverage of decedents; 1966–1968: information on the link between smoking and cancer mortality; and in 1986: data on comorbid conditions, disabilities, alcohol use, and access to healthcare services.
National Maternal and Infant Health Survey (NMIHS)	http://www.cdc.gov/nchs/nvss/nmihs.htm	The objective of NMIHS was to collect data needed by federal, state, and private researchers to study factors related to poor pregnancy outcomes, including low birth weight, stillbirth, infant illness, and infant death. The NMIHS provided data on socioeconomic and demographic characteristics of mothers, prenatal care, pregnancy history, occupational background, health status of mother and infant, and types and sources of medical care received. Data from the study may be used to evaluate factors affecting adverse outcomes of pregnancy.
Medicare and Medicaid Data	Centers for Medicare & Medicaid Services, https://www.cms.gov/home/rsds.asp	Medicare and Medicaid data is very rich and provides information on individual and aggregate data of providers and beneficiary, and individual level health information. Minimum data sets (MDS) are also available via Centers for Medicare and Medicaid services, and provide information for all residents at Medicaid- and Medicare-certified nursing and long-term care facilities.
Behavior Risk Factor Surveillance System (BRFSS)	CDC, http://www.cdc.gov/brfss/	The BRFSS is a state-based system of health surveys that collects information on health risk behaviors, preventive health practices, and healthcare access primarily related to chronic

(continued)

Table 8–3 List of Selected Publically Available Databases *(Cont'd)*

Database	Source	Brief description
		disease and injury. For many states, the BRFSS is the only available source of timely, accurate data on health-related behaviors. More than 350,000 adults are interviewed each year, making the BRFSS the largest telephone health survey in the world. States use BRFSS data to identify emerging health problems, establish and track health objectives, and develop and evaluate public health policies and programs. Many states also use BRFSS data to support health-related legislative efforts.
Youth Risk Behavior Surveillance System (YRBSS)	CDC, http://www.cdc.gov/HealthyYouth/yrbs/index.htm	The YRBSS monitors priority health-risk behaviors and the prevalence of obesity and asthma among youth and young adults. YRBSS monitors six categories of priority health-risk behaviors among youth and young adults, including behaviors that contribute to unintentional injuries and violence, tobacco use, alcohol and other drug use, sexual risk behaviors, unhealthy dietary behaviors, and physical inactivity. In addition, YRBSS monitors the prevalence of obesity and asthma.

Source: Adapted from Bibb, S. C. G. (2007). Issues associated with secondary analysis of population health data. *Applied Nursing Research, 20*, 94–99; and specific websites for datasets.

CONCLUSION

Concept measurement is a critical part of the research process. Measurement is the process of assigning values to concepts, objects, behaviors, and events according to a set of rules. Selecting the concepts of interest and then operationalizing the appropriate measures is an essential step in the research process. Care should be taken to minimize threats to measurement validity and reliability because the results of the research are only as good as the measures used in the studies. Whenever possible, it is wise to use measures and instruments developed and tested by previous researchers. This saves time and effort, as it avoids "reinventing the wheel." Newly created measures should be pilot tested and analyzed to test their reliability and validity.

Some of the common problems that may occur in data collection include biased sample selection, subject attrition, external unmeasured confounders, researcher biases, and errors made as a result of lack of training or skills in data collection techniques. Most of these problems can be avoided before data collection begins by knowing the lessons learned by previous researchers and anticipating as many potential problems as possible. Strategies for correctly collecting data and avoiding threats to validity and reliability should be clearly recorded in the study protocol. Then all members of the research team should be thoroughly trained according to the procedures in the protocol. Once the data is collected, they should be stored securely and separately from subject-identifying information to maintain the confidentiality of subject responses.

VOCABULARY

Conceptualization	Level of measurement	Reliability
Concurrent validity	Likert scales	Semantic differentials scales
Convergent validity	Operationalization	Semi-structured questions
Discriminant validity	Ordinal	Structured question
Internal consistency	Predictive validity	Survey
Inter-rater reliability	Rating scales	Test-retest reliability
Interval scales	Ratio scales	Validity

STUDY QUESTIONS AND EXERCISES

1. Give novel examples of variables with each of the four levels of measurement. With validity in mind, construct the relevant survey questions and response options.
2. Distinguish reliability and validity and explain how they can be measured. Include specific examples.
3. Describe the different methods of scale construction. Include specific examples of the different types.
4. Describe and give examples of the different methods of qualitative data collection.
5. Draft the data collection protocol for your particular study. Include information about data collection procedures, measures, tests for validity and reliability, and follow-up if relevant.
6. Read the abstract and methods section presented below. This article was published in 2009 in *International Electronic Journal of Health Education*, volume 12, pages 162–174. Use the information in this chapter and the abstract to answer the following questions:
   a. What instruments did the authors use to collect their data?
   b. Did they use survey or scales to collect their data?
   c. If a scale was used to collect data, what type of scale was it?
   d. How was validity or reliability measured in this study?

Exercise Self-Efficacy and Perceived Wellness Among College Students in a Basic Studies Course. Cara L. Sidman, BA, MS, PhD; Michelle Lee D'Abundo, PhD; Nancy Hritz, PhD.

Abstract

University basic studies courses provide a valuable opportunity for facilitating the knowledge, skills, and beliefs that develop healthy behaviors to last a lifetime. Belief in one's ability to participate in physical activity and exercise self-efficacy is a psychological construct that has had a documented impact on physical activity. Although previous research has investigated self-efficacy, physical activity, and wellness in various contexts, this study has specifically focused on exercise self-efficacy and perceived wellness in a college population. The purpose of the study was to determine the relationship between exercise self-efficacy and perceived wellness in a sample of college students enrolled in a basic studies physical activity and wellness course. After surveying 611 students, the results indicated that total exercise self-efficacy significantly predicted perceived wellness and the wellness subscales of physical, spiritual, intellectual, psychological, and emotional dimensions ($p < 0.05$). However, exercise self-efficacy did not significantly predict social wellness. These findings are of particular relevance because a predictive relationship between exercise self-efficacy and perceived wellness is in need of examination. This study indicated that development of exercise self-efficacy through strategically planned curricula and educational programs may be an effective way to improve wellness among college students.

Methods

Participants

A population of 1,037 students enrolled in a required mid-Atlantic coastal university basic studies course, *Physical Activity & Wellness* (PED 101), were invited to participate in the study during the Spring 2008 semester. The majority of the enrolled PED 101 students were sophomores (53%), followed by juniors (21%), seniors (19%), and freshmen (7%). Eighty-four percent were white and 54% were females.

This two-credit course focused on the development of knowledge, skills, and attitudes to facilitate health and wellness behaviors to last a lifetime. The course consisted of one lecture and two physical activity labs each week (students select their lab from a variety of activities).

Instrumentation

Following the demographic questions, the participants were directed to complete the Perceived Wellness Survey (PWS), a 36-item, self-administered, multidimensional questionnaire scored on a six-point Likert scale from 1, "Very strongly disagree," to 6, "Very strongly agree." This scale measures overall well-being on six dimensions— physical, social, emotional, intellectual, psychological, and spiritual—with six questions devoted to each dimension. Higher scores indicated greater total wellness overall and in each of the subscales. The instrument has shown construct validity and reliability in previous research, and has been used to assess college populations. Moreover, the items in the PWS were shown to have high internal reliability overall (alpha = 0.91) and consistency in the subscales. Sample items from each dimension include, "I am always optimistic about my future" (psychological), "I sometimes think I am a worthless individual" (emotional), "I will always seek out activities that challenge me to think and reason" (intellectual), "My friends will be there for me when I need help" (social), "My physical health is excellent" (physical), and "I believe that there is a real purpose for my life" (spiritual).

Participants were then directed to complete the Self-Efficacy and Exercise Habits Survey, which was used to assess the psychological construct of self-efficacy in the physical activity context. This 12-item questionnaire measured participants' confidence levels in motivating themselves to exercise consistently for at least 6 months. This survey was based on a 5-point Likert scale from "I know I cannot" (1) to "Maybe I can" (3) to "I know I can" (5). This scale was selected due to its simplicity, its previous validation on a similar undergraduate student population, and its established test-retest reliability and internal consistency.

REFERENCES

Babbie, E. (1990). *Survey research methods* (2nd ed.). Belmont, CA: Wadsworth.

Bibb, S. C. G. (2007). Issues associated with secondary analysis of population health data. *Applied Nursing Research, 20*, 94–99.

Boslaugh, S. (2007). *Secondary data sources for public health: A practical guide.* New York: Cambridge University Press.

Burns, N., & Grove, S. K. (2005). *The practice of nursing research: Conduct, critique, and utilization* (5th ed.). St. Louis, MO: Elsevier Saunders.

Centers for Disease Control and Prevention. (2012). Surveys and data collection systems. Retrieved January 10, 2012, from http://www.cdc.gov/nchs/surveys.htm.

Friis, R. H., & Sellers, T. A. (2009). *Epidemiology for public health practice* (4th ed.). Sudbury, MA: Jones & Bartlett.

Jenkins, C. D. (1966). The semantic differential for health. A technique for measuring. Beliefs about diseases. *Public Health Reports, 81*(6), 549–558.

Malhotra, N. K. (2006). Questionnaire design and scale development. In R. Grover & M. Vriens, (Eds.), *The handbook of marketing research: Uses, misuses, and future advances* (pp. 83–94). Thousand Oaks, CA: Sage Publications.

Monsen, E. R., & Van Horn, L. (2008). *Research successful approaches* (3rd ed.). Chicago, IL: American Dietetic Association.

Osgood, C. E., Suci, G. J., & Tannenbaum P. H. (1957). *The measurement of meaning.* Urbana, IL: University of Illinois.

Schneeweiss, S. (2007). Understanding secondary databases: A commentary on "Sources of Bias for Health State Characteristics in Secondary Databases." *Journal of Clinical Epidemiology, 60*(7), 648–650.

Stevens, S. S. (1946). On the theory of scales of measurement. *Science, 103*(2684), 677–680.

Weinstein, J. N., & Deyo, R. A. (2000). Clinical research: Issues in data collection. *SPINE, 25*(24), 3104–3109.

Analyzing Data

VIII. Vocabulary

IX. Study Questions and Exercises

We tend to regard statistics as though they are magical, as though they are more than mere numbers. We treat them as powerful representations of the truth; we act as though they distill the complexity and confusion of reality into simple facts.
—Joel Best, 2001, p. 160

INTRODUCTION

Our ethical responsibility as researchers does not end when the data are collected. Many consumers of our research are not statistically savvy. They sometimes "believe" without question the "truth" of our research. Peer review committees are mandated to prevent the publication of false or biased results, but why waste their time and our effort and money generating misleading or garbage results? The purpose of this chapter is to present the reader with information useful for choosing, conducting, and interpreting the results of appropriate statistical methods—methods that are best suited for particular research questions, study designs, measurements, and study samples.

It is assumed that the reader has at least an introductory background in statistics and biostatistics.[*] The details (i.e., formulas and calculations) are not the focus of this chapter. Many very good statistics and biostatistics textbooks and documentation for statistical packages (e.g., SPSS, SAS, and even Excel) are available for reference. Instead, the purpose of this chapter is to give directions that should help the reader navigate the options and limitations in research analysis. Data analysis packages such as SPSS and SAS are quite user-friendly. An analytic method can be run with the click of the mouse on a drop-down menu. The inappropriate use of methods and ignorance of necessary assumptions and limits leads to results that are not valid or useful. This chapter is intended to help the reader avoid these mistakes.

---

[*]For relevant background information, see Bush (2012); Chang (2011); Diggle & Chetwynd (2011); Gerstman (2008); Glantz (2011); Hebel & McCarter (2012); Källén (2011); Katz (2011); Lachin (2011); Merrill (2013); Rossi (2010); Sullivan (2012); Vittinghoff (2011).

FROM RAW DATA TO VARIABLES

Our data are collected. Now what? We need to "process" the data and create a computer-based data file to analyze. We may have a raw (i.e., ASCII) data file or a stack of papers. The latter form of data needs to be entered into a computerized data file. The former likely needs some cleaning and modification. As in every other step of the research process, validity is a primary concern in processing the raw data.

Data recorded by hand onto paper forms must be entered into a computer database. Data can be entered directly into a statistical analysis program or a basic format that can be converted to an analyzable format. The best practice for entering data by hand is to construct a data entry program with appropriate fields (e.g., alpha, numeric, number of decimal places) for each measure. Then a data clerk would enter all data from the forms into the program. Next, (ideally) another data entry clerk would enter the data again, called double-entry, and any discrepancies between the two entries would be compared to the hard copy data form to resolve the data entry error.

Data entered directly by the subject or an interviewer into an electronic file (i.e., Computer assisted self interview [CASI] using Survey Monkey online data collection) should also be checked for errors. However, many potential data entry errors can be avoided by programming range limits (an error message appears if a number outside a predetermined range is entered) and correct and logical skip patterns (if the root question does not apply to the subject, he or she is automatically skipped out of follow-up questions). The resulting data are only as good as the custom data entry file, so particular care should be taken to create a correct entry file. Test runs of data entry are key to determine bugs or errors that should be corrected before actual data collection commences.

Whether the data file is hand-entered or directly entered, additional checking or "cleaning" of the data should take place. Consistency checks correlate similar measures to check for illogical responses. For example, if a subject responds that he or she currently uses marijuana, but in another measure responds that he or she has used marijuana zero times in the past year, a discrepancy should be resolved. If hand-entered, the hard copy should be checked for clues about the discrepancy. With sufficient evidence and reasonable assumptions, the data can be corrected—either the subject would be coded as not being a current marijuana user, or may be imputed, for example, as the average number of times used in the past year for the sample as a whole. If out-of-range responses are possible and occur, these too should be resolved by checking the hard-copy data form and/or using other relevant data to make an educated guess about the correct response. Sometimes, the best correction for a too high numeric response is to change it to the highest possible and practical value.

Similar methods can be used to "impute" data that are missing (either skipped or refused). Information from similar measures can offer clues as to how the subject would have answered (or tested, etc.) if a response was entered for the item with missing data. An obvious imputation would be to change a missing value for the question about current marijuana use to an affirmative for a subject who said he or she used marijuana at least weekly during the past year. Imputation of missing data can have a considerable payoff in terms of statistical power because a case or subject with missing data on one of a number of variables in an analysis will be excluded from the entire analysis. Imputation is also important in studies with small samples. It is important to document all data changes and imputations in narrative form in the codebook (discussed shortly). Future use and users of the data may require different assumptions, or even no changes and imputations.

When data cleaning is complete, the raw data are organized into variables. The important thing about variables is that they vary. A variable has two or more categories across which subjects are distributed. There is variation across categories. A variable with three categories (say low, medium, high) should have proportions of the sample in each category. If 100% of subjects are in the "low" category, this is not a variable. We will discuss later how to "fix" variables with inadequate variation. First, we will illustrate the connection between raw data and variables in **Figure 9–1**.

The top table in Figure 9–1 shows a simple data-entry or raw data screen. It is in this screen or file that we make the corrections and imputations discussed above. Each row shows the responses for each subject on four separate measures—sex, race, cigarette smoking, and weight in pounds. For example, the first row is for the subject with ID number 01. The values indicate that subject 01 is a Caucasian male light smoker who weighs 180 pounds. The variables created from the four measures are shown in the small boxes. These are essentially a summation of each of the columns in the raw data file. Counting the Ms and Fs for sex, there are five males and five females as indicated in the frequency distribution for sex variable.

The race variable is an example of a variable with a potential variation problem. Fifty percent of the sample is Caucasian, 40% African American,

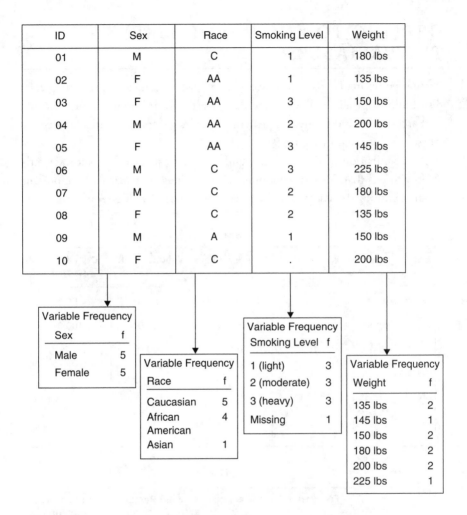

FIGURE 9–1 Raw Data to Variables

and only 10% Asian. We will discuss the problem with low variation variables and ways to treat them shortly. Notice there is missing data in the smoking variable. Subject number 10 refused to answer the question. Most statistical analysis packages show missing data with a period (.). Unless there is a logical and reasonable reason to recode this case (or subject response) as a smoker or non-smoker, then this case will be excluded from all analysis using the variable smoking status. So the sample size, or n for this variable would be nine rather than 10. We will discuss the weight variable shortly.

GETTING TO KNOW (AND LIKE) THE VARIABLES

At this point in the data processing, it is wise to run and print frequency distributions for all variables in the data set. The distributions should include both frequencies and relative frequencies (percentages) for each variable category. These are illustrated in **Figure 9–2**.

An examination of the frequency and relative frequencies can indicate variables with less than ideal distributions. Distributions are particularly important when examining the associations between two or more variables. A two-way table

Sex

	Frequency	Percent	Valid Percent	Cumulative Percent
Valid Male	5	50.0	50.0	50.0
Female	5	50.0	50.0	100.0
Total	10	100.0	100.0	
Missing	0	0.0		
Total	10	100.0		

Smoking Level

	Frequency	Percent	Valid Percent	Cumulative Percent
Valid 1	3	30.0	33.3	33.3
2	3	30.0	33.3	66.6
3	3	30.0	33.3	100.0
Total	9	90.0	100.0	
Missing	1	10.0		
Total	10	100.0		

FIGURE 9–2 Frequency Distributions

(one variable in the rows and the other in the columns) or especially multi-way tables with small (< 5) or empty cell frequencies result in unreliable measures of association between the variables. Similarly, variables with skewed distributions in which frequencies are relatively high at one end of the response range and very low at the other end need to be analyzed a particular way or recoded.

Examples of a problematic two-way table and a skewed distribution are presented in **Figure 9–3**. For these examples, assume our hypothetical study has a sample size of 100 rather than 10. As illustrated in Figure 9–3, the relatively small number of Asians in our example study results in cells that are too small and even empty cells in a two-way crosstabulation (crosstab). In addition, the skewed distribution of weight will limit the ability to use analytic techniques that require the ability to calculate means and standard deviations. (These issues will be discussed shortly.) The important point in this stage of data processing is that "problematic" variables may need to be modified or transformed in order to be analyzable.

Recoding Variables

Recoding variables can make them more analyzable by combining low-frequency response values with others and grouping or truncating skewed distributions. However, recoding decisions must be made in the context of conceptual issues specific to the study question and design. In our study example, combining Asians with Caucasians or with African Americans may or may not make sense given the focus of the study. Truncating the weight variable at 250 pounds (i.e., one category combining subjects weighing 250 and more pounds) may not make conceptual sense if the focus of the study is obese and morbidly obese persons. In addition, limiting the variability of a variable also limits the choice of analytic techniques that are appropriate (as discussed shortly).

Combining Categories

Technically, recoding a variable means changing the codes of its categories. Variables can be recoded using the DATA command in SAS (SAS, 2002–2003). This change is illustrated in **Figure 9–4**. For this example recode, the numeric codes for the categories are "1" for Caucasian, "2" for African American, and "3" for Asian. (Most packages assign numeric codes for alpha categories in the order they listed for the variable.) Recoding "3" into "1" combines the two categories. The exact labels for categories vary by statistical package, but this example shows that the remaining categories ("1" and "2" or "Else") should remain unchanged ("Same"). The first recoded variable is given a new name RACERC (RC for

Examples of Potentially Problematic Distributions
Race and Smoking Level Crosstabulation

			Smoking Level			
			Low	Moderate	Heavy	Total
RACE	Caucasian	Count	22	13	15	50
		% Within RACE	44.0%	26.0%	30.0%	100.0%
		% of Total	22.0%	13.0%	15.0%	50.0%
	African American	Count	20	15	5	40
		% Within RACE	50.0%	37.5%	12.5%	100.0%
		% of Total	20.0%	15.0%	5.0%	40.0%
	Asian	Count	8	2	0	10
		% Within RACE	80.0%	20.0%	0.0%	100.0%
		% of Total	8.0%	2.0%	0.0%	10.0%
Total		Count	50	30	20	100
		% Within RACE	50.0%	30.0%	20.0%	100.0%
		% of Total	50.0%	30.0%	20.0%	100.0%

WARNING: 33.3% of cells have counts ≤ 5.

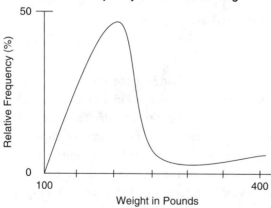

FIGURE 9–3 Examples of Potentially Problematic Distributions

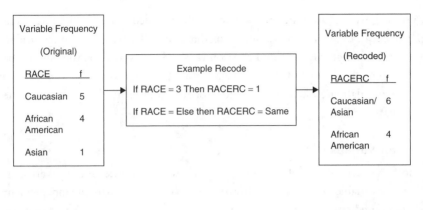

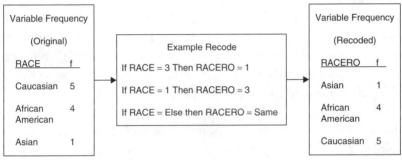

FIGURE 9–4 Examples of Variable Recoding

Recoded) to distinguish it from the original variable called RACE. It is important to always check the frequency distribution of the recoded variable to make sure the recode worked as intended.

Reordering Categories and Using Missing Data

It might also be necessary to reorder the categories of a variable. We will discuss the importance of this type of recoding when we cover scale creation a little later. The second example of recoding, RACERO (where RO stands for Reorder), changes category "1" to "3" and "3" to "1." Category "2" remains unchanged in the middle. It may also be appropriate, if it makes conceptual sense, to recode missing data into valid categories. For example, consider a variable measuring the last time the subject visited a physician. The categories are (1) more than one year ago, (2) within the past year, and (.) missing. One could make the argument that subjects who do not respond to this measure probably have not been to the doctor for some time. Consequently, the missing values (.) can be recoded into category "1." Any such recodes should be revealed in the resulting research paper, because they rely on assumptions that should be evaluated by the reader. If there is no arguable conceptual reason to recode missing data, they should be left as missing and excluded from the analysis. Variables with large proportions of missing data are likely invalid and probably should not be analyzed in the first place.

Dummy Variables

Another potential use of recoding procedures is to create dummy variables. Dummy variables are used in multivariable analysis (more than one independent variable predicting one dependent variable) to compare the effect of dummy group membership on the dependent variable. Dummy variables are typically coded as "0" and "1," and the "effect" on the dependent variable shows the numeric change in the dependent variable comparing category "1" to category "0." For example, an experimental study of the effect of a new drug on harmful cholesterol levels would code a dummy variable for experimental group where "1" is the new drug group and "0" is the control group. The dummy variable is included in a multivariable analysis (including potential confounding variables or simple covariates) predicting cholesterol level. The resulting numeric coefficient is interpreted as the difference in cholesterol level for the new drug compared to the control group.

Creating Scales

Sometimes important concepts are complex or multidimensional and cannot be measured by one variable. Consequently, it is necessary to create a multidimensional measure by combining individual variables into a scale. Scales are created using the DATA command in SAS. The most basic, and possibly most commonly used, scale is the Guttman (or Cumulative or Additive) Scale. A Guttman Scale is simply the summation of two or more variables. The resulting scale includes more than one dimension of the concept being represented, where each variable represents one dimension of the concept.

For example, stress is an important yet complex concept in the etiology of chronic diseases. Most of us hear the word "stress," and we think we know what it means. But how do we measure it in a way to represent truly what we mean by stress? In the late 1960s, social scientists Thomas Holmes and Richard Rahe (1967) developed the Social Readjustment Rating Scale after years of studying the concept of stress. The scale includes two dimensions of stress—frequency and seriousness of stressful events. These events, ranked from most to least severe, are:

1. Death of a spouse
2. Divorce
3. Marital separation
4. Incarceration
5. Death of a close family member
6. Personal injury or illness
7. Marriage
8. Job loss
9. Marital reconciliation
10. Retirement

Each event is weighted by relative severity and multiplied by the frequency of occurrence during a specified period of time, and these products are added to create the scale. The higher the value of the scale, the greater is the stress.

Individual variables should be examined carefully before using them to create a scale. Categories may need to be combined to make variables consistent in relative contribution to the scale. For example, it may be appropriate that each variable has four categories coded "0" to "3" so that a scale adding four such variables would have a range of "0" to "12." A variable with five categories would contribute more to the scale. Perhaps most importantly, individual variables to be added for a scale should all be coded in the same direction (low to high or high to low; "0" for No and "1" for Yes) so that the magnitude of the scale has conceptual meaning. High on the scale means high on the concept, or high on the scale means low on the construct. Consistency in the coding of individual variables is vital in the creation of meaningful scales. Once the scale is created, the frequency distribution of the new scale measure should be examined to ensure that the scale was created as intended.

Levels of Measurement

The data are cleaned, variables recoded, and scales created, so are we now ready to begin the analysis? Well, almost. At this point, we should examine the level of measurement of our variables because this dictates the types of analysis we can use appropriately. The measurement of our dependent variable is particularly important in choosing the correct analysis technique. The dependent variable is the outcome, the effect, or what is caused. The independent variables are the causes, confounders, or covariates (i.e., they covary to together affect the dependent variable when included in the same analytic model). For good measure, we will review the levels of measurement of variables beginning with the level with the most limited analytic techniques. Each level of measurement is illustrated in Figure 9–1.

Dichotomous and Categorical Variables

Categorical variables have qualitatively, but not quantitatively, meaningful response options. This class of variables is also known as nominal. A dichotomous variable is a categorical variable with two categories. The categories do not have an inherently meaningful numeric value. Sex is a dichotomous variable. It has two categories (male and female) that do not have meaningful numeric values. We stress the word "meaningful" because numeric values can be assigned to the categories for analytic purposes (e.g., dummy variables), but they do not inherently define the meaning of the categories. Other examples of dichotomous measures are: true/false, yes/no, urban/rural, and so on.

Race is an example of a categorical variable. The response options are qualitatively meaningful categories, and there are more than two categories. The distinction between dichotomous and categorical variables is important in choosing the appropriate analytic techniques. Like dichotomous variables, the response options of categorical variables cannot be ordered in any meaningful way. There is no consistent reason to rank Caucasian first, last, or in the middle of race categories. Other examples of categorical variables are never married/widowed/divorced/currently married, blue/green/gray/hazel/brown eye color, and so on.

Ordinal Variables

Ordinal variables have categories that can be ordered in a meaningful way. However, the categories do not have an intrinsic numeric value. The distance between categories is not meaningful. Education level is an example of an ordinal variable. Although there is a 1-year interval between grades 11 and 12, there is greater conceptual difference between completing grade 11 and completing grade 12 to graduate from high school. Similarly, a pain-severity scale from 1 (no pain) to 10 (unbearable pain) likely has a qualitatively different interval between 1 and 2 compared to that between 9 and 10. The ordinal example in Figure 9–1 is smoking level—light, moderate, and heavy. Without quantifying the frequency of smoking and the quantity of cigarettes smoked, these categories do not have meaningful intervals between them.

Likert response scales are also examples of ordinal measures. Likert scales typically have an odd number of response options ranging from one end of a continuum to the other. A common example is a measure of the level of agreement with some statement, say the ease of administration of an experimental drug: "I find it easy to fit the schedule of taking drug X into my usual daily routine: strongly disagree; disagree; neither disagree nor agree; agree; or strongly agree." Note that there is typically a middle category representing no opinion either way.

Continuous Variables

Continuous variables have categories with inherently meaningful numeric values. Our example of a continuous variable in Figure 9–1 is weight in pounds. The variable has a meaningful interval between categories (1 pound) and an absolute zero (0 pounds means no weight—on earth). Because an absolute zero grounds the scale of this variable, we can calculate meaningful ratios, where 200 pounds is twice that of 100 pounds. Hence, continuous variables with an absolute zero (where 0 means 0) are called ratio variables.

Interval measures are another type of continuous variable. The categories have meaningful numeric values; the intervals between categories are meaningful; but there is no absolute zero. Temperature in degrees Fahrenheit is an example of an interval variable. The interval between categories (1°) is meaningful, but 0°F does not mean the absence of temperature. The value 0°F is 1° higher than –1°F and 1° lower than positive 1°F. For this reason, it does not make sense to say 60°F is two times greater than 30°F. It does not make sense because the scale is not grounded with an absolute zero. In epidemiology, the majority of continuous variables are ratio rather than interval.

DESCRIBING THE DATA

Descriptive statistics are used to describe variables. A variable's features of interest are the range of values or categories, the number of subjects included in the variable, the distribution of subjects across categories of the variable, the average or typical variable category, and the degree of spread or dispersion of subjects across the range of categories. These statistics are useful in at least three ways: (1) They are study results themselves, (2) they can indicate potential selection and response bias, and (3) they determine the appropriate analytic use of the variable. Demonstrating that 80% of lifetime smokers develop emphysema, or that smokers who develop emphysema smoked, on average, for 32 years, are meaningful results using descriptive statistics. A random sample of adults in the United States with 40% African Americans suggests a selection or response problem. As discussed earlier, variables with small samples in some categories or with skewed distributions indicate the need for variable modification or the use of specific analytic techniques that address these weaknesses.

Variable Size and Distribution

The number of subjects included in a variable and their distribution across categories can be presented for variables at all levels of measurement. In fact, these are the only appropriate descriptive statistics for categorical and ordinal variables. Knowledge of the sample sizes in individual variables is important for two reasons: (1) A variable with a lot of missing data (small n compared to the overall sample n) can be an invalid measure of the concept it is intended to measure, and (2) the size of a variable helps ground the interpretation of statistical significance (recall that large samples have more statistical power than small samples). Frequency distributions are generated using the PROC FREQ command in SAS.

Tables

Examples of variable sizes and frequency distributions are presented in Figure 9–2. These results are shown in tabular form and include the variable size (total) and the distribution of subjects in absolute numbers (frequencies or counts), and relative frequencies or percentages of the total (including and not including missing cases in the total—percentage and valid percentage, respectively). The cumulative percentage is simply the addition of percentages down categories. The cumulative percentage is useful for giving a quick idea of the dispersion of subjects across categories.

Variable size and distribution can also be shown in tabular form for continuous variables, but the tables can be large and tedious for variables with many (e.g., 50) categories. Often it is more appropriate to present frequency tables of continuous variables, where categories are grouped (e.g., less than 5, 5 to 10, 11 to 15, 16 to 20, and more than 20) to render the table more manageable and readable. (Note: When grouping categories, be sure they are exhaustive—include all possibilities—and mutually exclusive—do not have overlap in values between categories. Less than 5 and more than 20 is exhaustive in including all possible low and high values. Categories 5 to 10 and 10 to 15 would NOT be mutually exclusive, because the value 10 can be legitimately included in both categories.) Continuous variables can also be described with statistics (discussed shortly) and graphically.

Graphs

Graphic presentations of variable characteristics are beneficial for showing relative frequencies for continuous variables with many categories. They also add visual interest to research papers and presentations. Graphs and charts can be generated in the PROC FREQ command in SAS. The appropriate type of graph depends on the level of measurement of the variable. **Figure 9–5** presents examples of different types

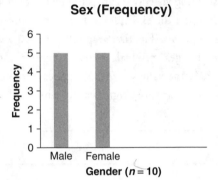

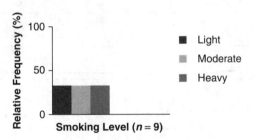

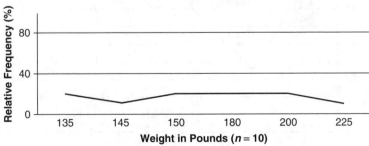

FIGURE 9–5 Graphic Presentation of Variable Size and Frequency Distribution

of graphs. Bar graphs (bars do not touch each other) are appropriate for categorical variables, because the categories have no relationship to each other. Pie charts are also suited for categorical variables. Histograms (with bars touching) are appropriate for ordinal variables, because there is a pattern or order in the categories (e.g., low to high). Line graphs are appropriate for continuous measures, because lines are an efficient way to represent a large number of categories with a meaningful numeric order.

Graphs can be misleading visually if care is not taken to choose the appropriate scale for the y-axis. Consider the examples in **Figure 9–6**. Both line graphs represent the exact same data points. The first graph illustrates a *Y* variable that is relatively rare or low and changes very little across categories of the *X* variable. The second graph, using the same values (of *X*, *Y*), appears to represent a *Y* variable with relatively high values that varies significantly with *X*. The proper scale for *Y*

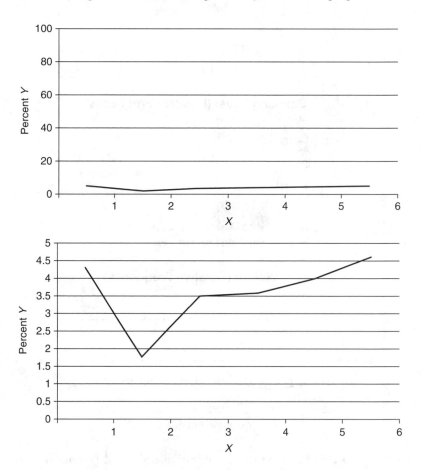

FIGURE 9–6 The Visual Impact of Differences in the Scale of the y-Axis

depends on the nature and relative magnitude of the values for X. Perhaps, the most important factor is the range of values of Y in the sample or population. If relatively small differences are significant or important (which will be determined by the focus of the study), then that scale should be adjusted to reflect the differences as large. Ratio values should be plotted on a log scale, which influences the visual impact of the graph. The point is to consider the importance of scale in reflecting a relationship graphically.

Measures of Central Tendency

Measures of central tendency can be calculated for variables of all levels of measurement, but only continuous variables can use all three—mean, median, and mode. Central tendency statistics are calculated using the PROC UNIVARIATE command in SAS. These measures indicate the average or typical value in the distribution of a variable. They utilize the numeric values of the variable categories in their calculations. The most well known and possibly most utilized is the mean or statistical average. The mean is simply the sum of all variable values (X) for all subjects divided by the number of subjects (n). For example, consider, again, the variable of WEIGHT introduced in Figure 9–1. The mean for this variable is (135 + 135 + 145 + 150 + 150 + 180 + 180 + 200 + 200 + 225)/10, or 1,700/10 = 170 pounds.

If the mean is so easy to calculate and understand, why do we need the median and the mode? There are two primary reasons: (1) A mean cannot be calculated meaningfully for categorical and ordinal variables, and (2) the shape of a frequency distribution for continuous variables may render the mean unreliable. More specifically, if there are extreme values or outliers on continuous variables, where a few subjects cluster on the highest or lowest values in the variable range, then the mean is unreliable. For example, say a few sumo wrestlers were included in our sample. They weighed 325, 360, and 410 pounds. Now, the mean is (135 + 135 + 145 + 150 + 150 + 180 + 180 + 200 + 200 + 225 + 325 + 360 + 410)/13, or 2,795/13 = 215 pounds. Note that the mean had been inflated by these extreme values (215 compared to 170). In this case, the median would be a better measure of central tendency. The median is the value below and above which 50% of the distribution lies. Consider the median for both distributions:

No sumo: 135 135 145 150 150 160 180 200 200 225

$$(150 + 160) / 2 = 155 = \text{Median}$$

With sumos: 135 135 145 150 150 180 180 200 200 225 325 360 410

Median

The median of 180 is closer in value to 155 than are the means of the distributions. To calculate the median by hand, the data should be arranged in order with every value (including repeated values) listed individually. If the sample size is an even number, the median is the average of the two middle values in the list. If the sample size is odd, the median is the middle value.

The median can be calculated for ordinal variables. Even though the categories do not have inherently meaningful numeric values, numbers can be assigned to categories for the purpose of calculating the median. Consider, again, our smoking level variable. The median is:

$$1 \; 1 \; 1 \; 2 \; \underset{\uparrow}{2} \; 2 \; 3 \; 3 \; 3$$
$$\text{Median}$$

We would not interpret the median as "2." We would interpret it in terms of the category represented by the value "2." Hence, the median smoking level in our sample is moderate.

The mode, or most common or frequent category, can be reported for continuous and ordinal variables. In addition, it is the only appropriate measure of central tendency for categorical variables. For our example variable RACE, Caucasian is the modal category (5 Caucasians compared to 4 African Americans and 1 Asian). An example of output of descriptive statistics is presented in **Table 9–1**. The standard deviation is discussed in the next section.

Measures of Dispersion

Measures of dispersion or variability indicate how "spread out" the subjects are across the range of variable categories. This measure coupled with the measure of central tendency gives us a very good idea of the frequency distribution of our variables. If we know the mean of our WEIGHT variable is 170 pounds and our measure of dispersion is small, then we know that the majority of subjects weigh around 170 pounds.

Table 9–1 Descriptive Statistics Output

		Descriptive Statistics			
	N	Minimum	Maximum	Mean	Standard deviation
Weight	10	135.00	225.00	170.00	31.45
Valid N	10				

The appropriate measures of dispersion for continuous variables are the variance and standard deviation. If a mean is reported, then variance and standard deviation should be reported. The variance is the average of the squared deviations of each data point (x) around the mean. The deviations are squared for mathematical reasons. The standard deviation is the square root of the variance. More specifically, the standard deviation is the square root ($\sqrt{}$) of the average ($/n-1$) squared deviations around the mean $[(x-\bar{X})^2 /]$. The standard deviation rather than the variance is typically reported because it is in the same scale as the variable. The smaller is the standard deviation value; the more compact is the dispersion of variable values around the mean.

The interquartile range is the measure of dispersion that should be reported for the median measure of central tendency. Again, the median is used with skewed continuous distributions (with outliers) and with ordinal variables. Where the median marks the variable value that separates the frequency distribution in half, the interquartile range marks the points where 25% of the distribution lies below and 25% lies above. In other words, the range represents the middle 50% of the distribution. Perhaps the best way to illustrate and present the median and interquartile range is with the Box-Whisker Plot. An example is presented in **Figure 9–7**. A quick view of the plot indicates that the values are fairly evenly distributed, with the median approximately in the middle of the range (Highest Actual Value to Lowest Actual Value). The box represents the interquartile range (75th percentile to 25th percentile). The median line would be lower for a distribution with outliers on the upper end of values (because the majority of cases are on the lower end) and higher for one with outliers on the lower end of values (most of the cases are on the higher end of variable values).

TESTING INFERENCES, RELATIONSHIPS, AND EFFECTS

Now, we get to the good stuff, the apex, the coup de gras, the big enchilada, the results—the answer to our research questions. These procedures have their own PROC command in SAS. The basic model tested in epidemiologic research is the relationship between an exposure and an outcome. Specific analytic models can be more or less complex than this basic model, but it provides the structure for most epidemiologic research. In this section, we will discuss analytic strategies appropriate for testing variations of this model. Consider the following example.

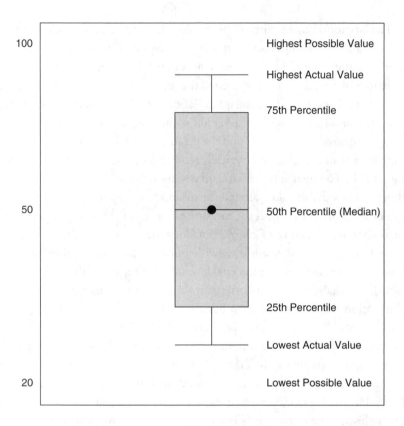

FIGURE 9–7 Example Box-Whisker Plot

Descriptive Study of Malignant Meningiomas in Upstate New York

"What is the prevalence of malignant meningiomas among adults in upstate New York in 2010?"

"What is the incidence of malignant meningiomas among adults in the 10 years from 2001 to 2010?"

"What patient characteristics are associated with malignant meningiomas?"

The first and third questions can be answered in a cross-sectional study. The second and third questions can be answered in a prospective cohort study. We will discuss appropriate analytic strategies for each question in turn. The appropriate analyses are summarized in **Table 9–2**.

What is the prevalence of malignant meningiomas among adults in upstate New York in 2010?

Table 9–2 Analytic Strategies for a Descriptive Study

Outcome measure	Level of measurement	Analysis goal	Calculation	Interpretation
Sample prevalence	Dichotomous	Estimate population prevalence	Confidence interval around estimate	The narrower the interval, the more precise the estimate
Sample prevalence	Dichotomous	Compare sample estimate to a national prevalence	Z or t hypothesis test	If the Z or t has a p-value ≤ 0.05 then the difference is statistically significant
Sample prevalence	Dichotomous	Test relationships between person-place-time characteristics and prevalence	Risk ratio or risk difference Z or t hypothesis test (correlate variable is dichotomous) Chi-square test of independence (correlate is categorical or ordinal)	If Z, t, or chi-square value has a p-value ≤ 0.05 then relationship is statistically significant
Sample incidence	Dichotomous	Estimate population incidence	Confidence interval around estimate	The narrower the interval, the more precise the estimate
Sample incidence	Dichotomous	Compare sample estimate to a national incidence	Z or t hypothesis test	If the Z or t has a p-value ≤ 0.05 then the difference is statistically significant
Sample incidence	Dichotomous	Test relationships between person-place-time characteristics and incidence	Risk ratio or risk difference Z or t hypothesis test (correlate variable is dichotomous) Chi-square test of independence (correlate is categorical or ordinal)	If Z, t, or chi-square value has a p-value ≤ 0.05 then relationship is statistically significant

(continued)

Table 9–2 Analytic Strategies for a Descriptive Study *(Cont'd)*

Outcome measure	Level of measurement	Analysis goal	Calculation	Interpretation
Test score	Continuous	Estimate the average test score	Confidence interval around the mean	The narrower the interval, the more precise the estimate
Test score	Continuous	Compare sample mean to a national mean	Z or t hypothesis test	If the Z or t has a p-value ≤ 0.05 then the difference is statistically significant
Test score	Continuous	Test relationships between person-place-time characteristics and test score	Difference in means Z or t hypothesis test (correlate is dichotomous) Analysis of variance (ANOVA) F statistic (correlate is categorical or ordinal)	If Z, t, or F value has a p-value ≤ 0.05 then relationship is statistically significant

Estimates and Confidence Intervals

A randomized sample of oncology practices is asked to provide the number and characteristics of patients with this type of tumor. Prevalence is calculated by dividing the number of patients (x) by the total size of the adult population in upstate New York ($\hat{p} = x / n$). A 95% confidence interval (CI) should be calculated to indicate the precision of our prevalence in estimating the true target population prevalence. We wish to infer the population parameter from our sample statistic, and we want to determine the precision of our inference.

$$95\% \ \text{CI} = \hat{p} \pm Z \sqrt{[\hat{p}(1-\hat{p})]/n}$$

where Z is the standardized value associated with 0.95 probability (e.g., 1.96) and n is the sample size. The confidence interval is one value below and one value above the prevalence estimate, indicating that we are 95% confident that the true population prevalence is within this interval. The narrower is the interval, the more precise is the estimate. A large sample size helps to assure a narrow interval.

We are also interested in comparing the prevalence in our study to the current national prevalence or an earlier prevalence for upstate New York. We find a difference when we subtract the national prevalence from our prevalence, but we want to know if the difference is statistically significant. We conduct a hypothesis test using Z or t as test statistics. A Z-score is used for larger samples ($n \geq 30$), and a t-score is appropriate for smaller samples ($n < 30$). To test the hypothesis that the prevalences are not equal (two-tailed test) or one is greater than the other (one-tailed test), we (or our statistical package) calculate the Z or t and determine the probability value associated with the score. The calculation is:

$$Z \text{ or } t = (\hat{p}_{sample} - \hat{p}_{comparison}) / \sqrt{\hat{p}_{comparison}(1 - \hat{p}_{comparison}) / n}$$

There are two ways we can determine if the Z or t is significant. First, we can set the critical probability or α to a level, usually 0.05. If our calculated value has a probability less than 0.05, the difference is statistically significant. Second, we can examine the actual p-value of our score and interpret its exact level of significance. The important distinction between α and p-value is the former is a preset threshold we wish to be below (0.05), and the latter is the exact probability value of the calculated Z or t.

Procedures for calculating confidence intervals and testing hypotheses are the same for estimating incidence. Incidence is calculated by dividing the number of new cases of malignant meningioma reported from January 1, 2000, to December 31, 2010, by the population size of those without the tumors on January 1, 2000. Like prevalence, incidence is a proportion that is treated as a dichotomous variable in analyses.

Associations

Another goal of descriptive epidemiology is to determine the relevant correlates of the prevalence or incidence of disease or disorder. The potential correlates measure characteristics of person, place, and time. The specific hypothesis test statistic depends on the level of measurement of the potential correlate. For a dichotomous person-characteristic such as sex, risk ratios or risk differences are calculated. Because sex is a nominal categorical measure, the order of comparison does not matter. An example risk ratio would measure the prevalence of tumors among women divided by the prevalence for men. A ratio greater than one (1) means that women have a higher prevalence than men, and the opposite is true for ratios less than one (1). A ratio of one (1) means that the prevalences are equal or there is no difference by gender. The risk difference measures the mathematical difference between two prevalences (or incidences). Again, the order does not matter. If we subtract the prevalence for men from that of women, a positive number would indicate that the prevalence for women is greater than that for men. A negative value means the opposite. A value of zero (0) means no difference in prevalences.

For risk ratios and differences that indicate a difference in prevalence (or incidence) between genders, we wish to test if the difference is large enough to be statistically significant. There are two ways to test for statistical significance. The first method is to calculate appropriate confidence intervals around the risk ratio or difference. If the confidence interval around the ratio includes the value one (1), then the difference is not statistically significant. If the interval around the risk difference includes zero (0), then the difference is not statistically significant. For example, the confidence interval for the risk difference would be:

$$95\% \text{ CI} = (\hat{p}_{female} - \hat{p}_{male}) \pm Z \sqrt{\frac{[\hat{p}_{female}(1 - \hat{p}_{female})]}{n_{female}} + \frac{[\hat{p}_{male}(1 - \hat{p}_{male})]}{n_{male}}}$$

The second method to test statistical significance of ratios or differences is to calculate the appropriate Z or t and test the hypothesis that the prevalences are different (two-tailed test) or that one is greater than the other (one-tailed test). The formula for risk difference is:

$$Z = (\hat{p}_{female} - \hat{p}_{male}) / \sqrt{\hat{p}_{overall}(1 - \hat{p}_{overall})\left(\frac{1}{n_{female}} + \frac{1}{n_{male}}\right)}$$

where the overall $\hat{p}$ is the prevalence for females and males combined. If the p-value is ≤ 0.05, then the difference is statistically significant.

If the potential correlate is categorical or ordinal (i.e., more than just two categories), then the chi-square test of independence is used to test for statistical significance of any differences. For example, say we want to compare the prevalence of tumors for urban, suburban, and rural areas of upstate New York. We group patients by either place of residence or place of treatment according to a definition of urban, suburban, and rural. We calculate the three prevalences and see that they are not equal to each other, but are the differences statistically significant? We calculate a chi-square test of independence to test for statistical significance. The structure of this test statistic is to compare the observed two-way cell frequencies to the frequencies that would be expected if there is no relationship between area of residence and prevalence, if there is no difference in the prevalences for urban, suburban, and rural. If the difference between the observed and expected cell frequencies is statistically significant, then the variables are associated with one another.

The chi-square test is calculated using the PROC FREQ command in SAS. The procedure creates a two-way table showing the frequencies of subjects in combinations of categories for both variables. An example is shown in Figure 9–3. For the area of residence by prevalence crosstab, area should be the row variable, and prevalence the column variable. The column variable is typically the outcome or dependent variable. Appropriate options to select include row percentages, expected frequencies, and chi-square. To interpret the relationship shown in the table, row percentages should be compared down columns. Essentially, the percentages of urban, suburban, and rural residents with malignant meningiomas are compared. If the calculated chi-square (usually called the Pearson chi-square) is significant, then there is a relationship between residence and prevalence.

The idea is the same, but the specific procedures for estimation and hypothesis testing are different for continuous outcomes. Rather than calculating and comparing proportions, means are compared. Say in our hypothetical study of malignant meningiomas, we use a hypothetical screening test ranging from 0 to 10, with higher scores meaning a higher likelihood of having a malignant meningioma. Assuming the distribution is fairly normal in shape (e.g., bell-shaped with the mean, median, and mode in the middle of the variable range), analyzing the means is appropriate. (We will talk about analyzing continuous variables with outliers/skewed distributions shortly.)

Similar to the analysis of proportions, evaluating the sample mean as an estimate of the target population mean requires the calculation of a confidence interval. However, the formula is different.

$$95\% \text{ CI} = \bar{X} \pm Z \frac{s}{\sqrt{n}}$$

where $\bar{X}$ is the sample mean and s is the standard deviation. Again, the narrower is the interval, the more precise is the estimate.

The calculation of Z (larger sample) or t (smaller sample) to compare the sample mean test score to a national mean uses the following formula:

$$Z = (\bar{X} - \mu) / (s / \sqrt{n})$$

where μ is the national or comparison mean.

If we want to compare the sample means for a dichotomous variable such as gender, the formula for Z or t is:

$$Z = (\bar{X}_{female} - \bar{X}_{male}) / (S_p \sqrt{\frac{1}{n_{female}} + \frac{1}{n_{male}}})$$

where S_p is the pooled standard deviation calculated by combining the group (female and male) standard deviations and sample sizes. To compare two means using SAS, the PROC TTEST command provides the options for one- and two-group mean comparisons.

To compare means for ordinal or categorical measures, we use Analysis of Variance (ANOVA) and the F test statistic in the PROC GLM (general linear model) command in SAS. For example, we may want to compare the test score means for urban, suburban, and rural patients. With ANOVA we can compare more than two means to one another simultaneously. The F statistic is calculated by analyzing the variations of the data around the overall mean and each group (or category) mean. Biostatistics textbooks (such as Sullivan, 2012) provide the formulas for calculating F by hand. The calculation for even the simplest ANOVA is tedious and time-consuming. Statistical packages, namely SAS, calculate F with the PROC GLM command. An example of an ANOVA printout is presented in **Table 9–3**. The sum of squares between groups is the deviation of group means around the overall mean. The sum of squares within groups is the variation of each x value around its group mean. The degrees of freedom (df) for between groups is the number of means being compared (k) minus one (1) or ($3 - 1 = 2$). The df for within groups is sample size (N) minus the number of means being compared (k) or ($100 - 3 = 97$). The mean squares are the sums of squares divided by their respective df. The F statistic is the mean squares between groups divided by the mean squares within groups. The higher is the value of F, the lower is the p-value (sig.) or the greater the statistical significance. Again, a larger sample is more likely to yield a statistically significant F.

Table 9–3 Sample ANOVA Output

	Test score				
	Sum of squares	df	Mean square	F	Sig.
Between groups	310.3	2	155.2	67.5	0.000
Within groups	220.8	97	2.3		
Total	531.1	99			

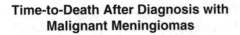

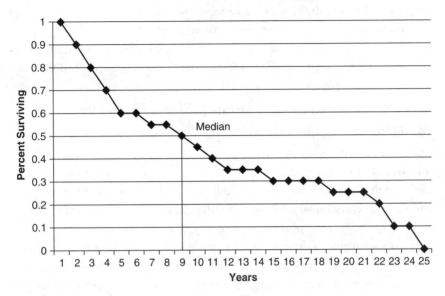

FIGURE 9–8 Example Kaplan-Meier Survival Curve

Survival Analysis

Another descriptive analytic technique commonly used in epidemiologic research is survival analysis.* Survival analysis can also be causal, as we will discuss in the next section. As a descriptive analysis staying in the theme of our example study, a relevant research question is: "What is the median survival time of patients diagnosed with malignant meningiomas?" In this case, the outcome variable is time-to-event. A survival function represents the probability that a subject survives past a certain time point. In SAS, survival analysis is found in the PROC LIFETEST and PROC PHREG commands. There are a few estimation options for survival functions. The Kaplan-Meier approach to survival analysis is a popular method in epidemiology.

The Kaplan-Meier approach recalculates the survival probability each time an event occurs (i.e., each time a subject passes away or drops out of the study). An example Kaplan-Meier survival curve is presented in **Figure 9–8**. The curve begins

---

*For more details about this technique see Allison (1995); Cox and Oakes (1984); Kleinbaum and Klein (2005); Lee and Wang (2003); Selvin (2008); Sullivan (2012).

at value one (1) on the *Y*-axis because all patients are alive at the beginning of the study period. The curve is fairly steep suggesting a relatively brief survival time after diagnosis. After 9 years, 50% of the patients had passed away. This is the median survival time. By year 25, everyone has passed away. We can conclude from this study, that the average survival time after diagnosis with malignant meningiomas is 9 years, and that the probability of survival past a quarter century is null.

Causal Relationships (Univariate): Single Predictors of Malignant Meningiomas

Statistical procedures for determining causal relationships between an exposure and an outcome are essentially the same as the few correlation procedures discussed in the previous section (i.e., risk differences and ANOVA). What makes the procedure a test of causal relationships is the satisfaction of some of the assumptions of causality. Perhaps most importantly, the exposure must occur in time before the outcome. Therefore, studies that can demonstrate that the exposure occurred before the outcome can test causal relationships. Case-control, cohort, and experimental studies are designed to demonstrate this temporal ordering or causal sequence. Again, the appropriate analytic procedure depends largely on the level of measurement of the outcome variable. In addition, for continuous outcomes, the appropriate procedure depends on whether or not the frequency distribution is normal in shape. This distinction will be discussed shortly.

A univariate relationship refers to the association between one outcome or dependent variable and only one exposure or independent variable. Statistics that measure the strength and statistical significance of this relationship are called, collectively, measures of association. Assuming the relationship is plausible, to be considered a causal relationship, the independent variable must precede the dependent variable. If the temporal order cannot be demonstrated, then a significant relationship should be interpreted as a correlation or association. For purposes of discussion, our causal questions are: "Is cell phone use related to incident malignant meningiomas?" and "Does drug X slow the rate of growth of malignant meningiomas?"

Cohort and Case-Control Study Analysis

Beginning with the first research question, there are a number of ways to address it analytically. The correct method depends, in part, on the study design and the level of measurement of the outcome and the exposure. For analyses with continuous outcomes, the appropriate analytic procedure depends on whether or not the outcome distribution is or can be assumed to be normal in shape. The univariate analytic procedures are outlined in **Table 9–4**. This list of analytic strategies may seem a bit daunting with many of the techniques named after statisticians with unusual names and the correct choice depending on a number of factors. However, if we systematically evaluate various features of our study and data, we can zero in on the one or few appropriate techniques. Then we should study up on the details (e.g., formulas, assumptions about the test statistic, and correct interpretations) of the specific appropriate procedure. The list in Table 9–4 touches on the most widely used procedures, but it is not exhaustive by any means.

Table 9–4 Analytic Strategies for Testing Univariate Causal Relationships

Exposure variable	Outcome variable			
	Prevalence or incidence (dichotomous)	Stage of tumor (ordinal)	Hypothetical test score (continuous)	
			Large sample/ normal distribution	Small sample/ non-normal distribution
Cell phone: no use/use (dichotomous)	Compare 2 proportions with risk difference, risk ratio, odds ratio (Z or t)	Compare 2 medians (Mann-Whitney U)	Compare 2 means (Z or t)	Compare 2 medians (Mann-Whitney U)
	Simple logistic regression (regression coefficient, odds ratio)		Simple linear regression (regression coefficient, R-squared)	
Cell phone use: never, some-times, always (ordinal)	Compare > 2 proportions (chi-square test of independence)	Compare > 2 medians (Kruskall-Wallis H)	Compare > 2 means (one-way ANOVA and F)	Compare > 2 medians (Kruskall-Wallis H)
	Simple logistic regression (regression coefficient, odds ratio)	Spearman correlation coefficient	Simple linear regression (regression coefficient, R-squared)	
Number of cell phone calls made in a typical week (continuous)			Pearson correlation coefficient	
			Simple linear regression (regression coefficient, R-squared)	

In choosing the proper technique, the most important first consideration is the level of measurement of the outcome. For dichotomous outcomes, we need to consider the study design. For case-control studies, the odds ratio is the only appropriate measure. The odds ratio compares the odds of having been exposed for cases relative to controls. The odds ratio is a ratio of two odds—one for each group being compared. Each odd is calculated by dividing the proportion of, say, individuals with a tumor who use cell phones by the proportion of those with a tumor who do not use cell phones. This odd (for the cases) is then divided by the similar odd for those without a tumor (the controls). Because the measure is a ratio, it is interpreted essentially the same way as the risk ratio discussed earlier. The formula, in words, looks like this:

$$OR = \frac{\left(P_{\text{tumor—cell phone use}} \ / \ P_{\text{tumor—no cell phone use}} \right)}{\left(P_{\text{no tumor—cell phone use}} \ / \ P_{\text{no tumor—no cell phone use}} \right)}$$

All three measures of association (odds ratio, risk difference, and risk ratio) can be used in the other study designs. Studies with continuous outcomes must investigate the distribution of the outcome variable. If it is normal in shape and/ or has a large sample size (the exact sample requirement depends on a number of factors), then means can be compared with one-way ANOVA (called one-way when only one independent variable is analyzed).

If these assumptions are not met, then nonparametric techniques (so named because a population parameter is not being estimated) must be used to compare median values. (Recall that the median is the appropriate measure of central tendency for skewed distributions.) Nonparametric techniques are also used with categorical and ordinal outcomes where the median is the appropriate measure of central tendency. Essentially, these techniques do not use actual variable data values to calculate test statistics. Instead, responses are "ranked" in order from lowest to highest, and values are assigned to the rankings ([1 to n]; means are used in the case of ties). Due to this ranking approach, these techniques are sometimes called "rank-order" procedures. Nonparametric procedures include Mann-Whitney U for comparing two medians, and Kruskall-Wallis H for comparing more than two medians. These procedures would be used in the analyses of the stage of cancer outcome or a skewed test score outcome. They can be found in the PROC UNIVARIATE command in SAS.

Two types of correlation coefficients and regression analyses are also included in Table 9–4. The appropriate types depend on the level of measurement of the outcome variable. Beginning with correlation methods, a correlation measures the relationship between two variables. The formulas indicate how closely the two variables vary together. Values range from −1.0 (perfect negative association) to +1.0 (perfect positive association). Correlation of 0.0 indicates no linear relationship between the two measures—they do not vary together in a linear pattern. A negative relationship is one in which one variable decreases as the other increases in category value. They covary in opposite directions. For example, a person's cholesterol level decreases as consumption of oats increases. Variables that covary in the same direction have a positive correlation. They can vary together in a positive direction or in a negative direction. As one increases, the other increases. As one decreases, the other decreases. A person's body weight increases with increasing fat consumption, and weight decreases with a decrease in fat consumption. (Note that this type of correlation indicates a dose-response relationship.) The higher is the value of the positive correlation and the lower is the value of the negative correlation, the stronger is the relationship. The statistical significance of a correlation value is tested by calculating p-values or confidence intervals. Confidence intervals that do not include the value zero (0) and p-values ≤ 0.05 indicate statistical significance.

A strong correlation and a dose-response relationship are two criteria for demonstrating causality. However, causality in a correlation can only be argued if (1) one variable measures an event that occurs, in time, before the other variable, and (2) a causal mechanism is plausible. Risk difference, risk ratios, and odds ratios are measures of correlation with dichotomous outcomes (and dichotomous exposures). Spearman correlations are appropriate for ordinal outcomes, and Pearson correlations are calculated for continuous outcomes. These procedures are found in the PROC FREQ and PROC CORR commands in SAS.

Simple regression methods are better representations of causal relationships than correlations because the independent and dependent variables are clearly delineated. Values of the dependent variable (Y) are "predicted" by those of the independent variable (X). The dependent variable is "dependent" on the independent variable. Again, the independent variable must measure an event that occurs before that measured in the dependent variable. Regression methods are better conceptual measures of causal relationships, but it should be noted that the correlation coefficients in simple regression models are equal to two-way correlation coefficients. The strength of regression analysis compared to correlations is especially relevant in multiple regression models (i.e., with more than one independent variable). These are discussed shortly.

Linear regression is used with continuous dependent variables. We begin discussing linear regression because it is a good introduction to regression analysis as it is relatively easy to understand conceptually. It is called "linear" regression because, with a continuous dependent variable, the relationship between the outcome and exposure can be graphed with a line or in a linear fashion. Values of the outcome (Y) can be plotted on a graph with knowledge of values of the exposure (X). The simple linear regression equation is:

$$\hat{Y} = b_0 + b_1 X_1$$

where $\hat{Y}$ is the dependent variable value, b_0 is the intercept value of Y when X is zero (0), X is the independent variable value, and b_1 is the slope or the change in Y with each unit change in X. The equation is shown graphically in **Figure 9–9**. The graph shows a positive relationship between frequency of cell phone use and a hypothetical continuously measured tumor test score. The individual data points are represented by the black circles. They show the value of both x and y for each individual subject. The joint values of the regression line are plotted by the regression equation. The values for b_0 and b_1 are calculated to minimize the squared deviations between the points and the line. The purpose of the line is to best represent the pattern of the combined (x and y) data points. The intercept (b_0) is the value of Y when X is zero (0). It is the starting point for the regression line. The slope (b_1) is the amount of change in Y with each unit change in X.

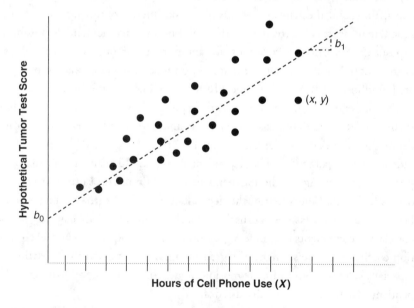

FIGURE 9–9 Regression Relationship Between Number of Hours of Cell Phone Use and Hypothetical Tumor Test Score

The larger is the value of the b_1 (relative to the scale of Y), the steeper is the slope of the regression line. The slope is also called the regression coefficient. The statistical significance of the regression coefficient is tested with a Z test or t test. P-values ≤ 0.05 are usually considered statistically significant. With linear regression, we can also calculate the R-square value, which indicates the percentage of the variation in the outcome that is explained by the exposure. For example, an R-square of 0.68 indicates that 68% of the variation in the outcome is explained by the exposure. The greater is the R-square, the more effective is the predictive model.

Logistic regression analysis is used with dichotomous dependent variables. Because the outcome is dichotomous, the regression coefficients (after some transformation) are interpreted as odds ratios comparing the odds of cell phone use relative to no cell phone use for the groups defined by the outcome variable (i.e., those with a tumor compared to those without). The simple logistic regression equation is:

$$\ln[\,p/(1-p)\,] = b_0 + b_1 x_1$$

where ln is the natural log of the odds of the dependent variable, b_0 is the intercept, and b_1 is the regression coefficient. The resulting regression coefficient is interpreted as an odds ratio when it is recalculated as its exponent. The independent or exposure measure is most easily interpreted when it is coded as a dummy variable (described earlier in this chapter) where the exposed group is coded "1" and the unexposed group is coded "0." The coefficient in this case is interpreted as the odds of the outcome when moving from 0 to 1 on, from unexposed to exposed, on the independent variable. Odds ratios for continuous independent variables indicate the odds of the outcome with each unit increase in X. For example, an odds ratio for tumor status with age (in single years) as an independent variable indicates the odds of having a tumor with each 1-year increase in age. The statistical significance of logistic regression coefficients is tested with the chi-squared test statistic.

Experimental Study Analysis

We will now move on to the second causal research question: "Does drug X slow the growth of malignant meningiomas?" This question requires an experimental study design. A study sample of subjects with the tumors is randomly assigned to the experimental group (drug X) or the control group (standard treatment). Pretest and posttest measures of tumor size are recorded and compared. The research hypothesis is that the mean reduction in tumor size is greater for the experimental group than for the control group. This design requires the use of statistical tests for dependent or matched groups. Each subject has two data points, so the method must address the fact that the data points are not independent of one another. An example using our hypothetical experimental study is presented in **Figure 9–10**. For this analysis, dependent group procedures are used to test the statistical significance of the mean reduction in tumor size for the control group and the experimental group separately. The analysis tests the significance of the mean of the difference from baseline (before intervention) to follow-up 6 months later. The formula is:

$$Z \text{ or } t = (\overline{X}_d - \mu_d) / (s_d / \sqrt{n})$$

where $\overline{X}_d$ is the observed mean of the difference from baseline to follow-up, μ_d is the mean of no difference or zero (0), and s_d is the standard deviation of the mean of the differences. We use t because our total sample n is only 12. The results show that there is a significant reduction in tumor size for drug X, but not for treatment as usual. However, a comparison of the two means of the differences is not statistically significant. We can conclude that drug X does reduce tumor size, but no better than does treatment as usual.

Survival Analysis

We can also examine whether an independent variable has an effect on survival functions, such as time-to-death after tumor diagnosis (discussed earlier and illustrated in Figure 9–8). Say we want to see if drug X extends survival time after tumor diagnosis more than does standard treatment. For this analysis, we use Cox proportional hazards regression analysis. This procedure can be found in PROC PHREG procedure in SAS.

Although still technically a type of survival analysis, Cox proportional hazards regression uses hazard rates rather than survival functions as the outcome measure. The distinction is subtle but important in the interpretation of results. Survival functions measure the probability that an individual survives (i.e., does not experience the event of death) past a certain time as a function of time. Hazard rates, on the other hand, measure the probability that an individual suffers the event of interest (i.e., death) conditional on the fact that he or she has survived up to a specific time. Simply put, a survival function is the probability that one survives as a function of time, while a hazard rate is the probability of not surviving as a function of having survived so far.

Tumor Size (cm)

Control Group (Standard Treatment)

Baseline	6-Month Follow-Up	Difference
1.2	0.8	−0.4
2.8	1.1	−1.7
0.9	0.8	−0.1
3.1	1.9	−1.2
1.6	0.6	−1.0
2.3	1.1	−1.2

$$\Sigma = -5.6$$
$$\bar{X} = -5.6/6 = -0.9$$

Is −0.9 statistically significant? $t = -0.9/(2.4/\sqrt{6}) = -0.19\ (p > 0.05)$ **NO**

Experimental Group (Drug X)

Baseline	6-Month Follow-Up	Difference
2.4	0.1	−2.3
1.9	0.0	−1.9
0.8	0.0	−0.8
3.3	0.2	−3.1
2.7	0.3	−2.4
	0.1	−1.4

$$\Sigma = -11.9$$
$$\bar{X} = -11.9/6 = -2.0$$

Is −2.0 statistically significant? $t = -2.0/(0.8/\sqrt{6}) = -16.7\ (p < 0.001)$ **YES**

Is there a statistically significant difference between the mean reduction for the control group and the mean reduction for the experimental group?

$$t = [-2.0 - (-0.9)]/1.6\sqrt{\frac{1}{5} + \frac{1}{5}} = -1.1/0.9 = -1.2\ (p > 0.05)\ \textbf{NO}$$

Conclusion: There is a significant mean reduction in tumor size in the experimental group but no significant mean reduction in the control group. The mean reductions in the experimental and control groups are not significantly different from each other. Drug X does reduce the size of tumors, but not significantly more than treatment as usual.

FIGURE 9–10 Analysis of the Effect of Drug X on Tumor Size

The hazard for a group (rather than a hazard rate) is the expected number of events (i.e., deaths) per unit of time. The calculation of the hazard ratio (the test statistic) uses the chi-square technique of comparing the number of observed events to the number that would be expected if the exposure and outcome are unrelated. The ratio is interpreted as the time to observed events relative to the time to expected events for the exposed group compared to that for the unexposed group—the ratio of the experimental relative to the control group. For example, say we calculate a hazard ratio of 5.23 for our experimental test of the effect of drug X on survival time. This would mean that the time until death is 5.23 times higher for patients who took drug X compared to those who had treatment as usual. The statistical significance of the hazard ratio is also calculated and interpreted.

Causal Relationship (Multivariable)

Multivariable analysis calculates the simultaneous effect of more than one variable (i.e., an exposure and several control variables) on the outcome. The regression coefficient for the effect of the exposure on the outcome is "adjusted" with the effects of the control variables. To better understand the purpose and interpretation of multivariable analysis, let us review the concepts of confounding and effect modification.

A relationship between an exposure and an outcome is confounded by some third factor (the confounder) if this third factor has significant effects on both the exposure and the outcome. The effect of the exposure on the outcome is really a function of the effect of the confounder on both variables. Confounding is a bias, a mistaken relationship. We need to discover it and, if present, adjust for it.

We can determine if confounding is present by conducting two hypothesis tests. The first test is for a significant relationship between the confounder and the exposure. The second test is for a relationship between the confounder and outcome. If both relationships are significant, confounding is present. If present, there are two general methods for adjusting for the effect of the confounder in the relationship between the exposure and outcome.

Cochran-Mantel-Haenszel Method

First is the Cochran-Mantel-Haenszel (CMH) method. This method is appropriate for dichotomous exposures and outcomes and a dichotomous or categorical confounder, and the procedure is found in the PROC FREQ command in SAS. Because the outcome is dichotomous, the measure of association is either risk ratio or odds ratio, depending on the study design. The CMH method calculates a risk or odds ratio that is a weighted average of the separate ratios that would be calculated for each category of the confounding variable. For example, a study examining risk factors for throat cancer due to cigar smoking showed that men who are bald are more likely to smoke cigars compared to men with a full head of hair. The investigators presumed that the men's age confounded this relationship, and they did find that older men were both more likely to be bald and to smoke cigars. Consequently, they calculated and reported a risk ratio that averaged the effect of baldness on throat cancer for young men and the effect for older men. The average is weighted by the relative group sizes of the young and old groups and the strength of association between exposure and outcome in the two age groups. Say the risk ratio between baldness and cancer without consideration of age (called the crude relationship) is 3.2, indicating that the risk is three times greater for bald men than for men with hair. However, the CMH risk ratio adjusting for age is only 1.2, suggesting virtually no difference in risk by baldness. This reduction in the ratio from crude to adjusted demonstrates and adjusts for confounding by age.

Multivariable Regression Models

Multivariable linear and logistic regression analyses can also adjust for confounding. The effects of multiple confounders can be adjusted simultaneously. (Linear regression is conducted using the PROC REG and logistic regression in the PROC LOGISTIC commands in SAS.) This adjustment method is commonly referred to as "controlling for the effects of other independent variables." The goal is to show the "true" effect of the exposure on the outcome, controlling for the effect of potential confounders and covariates. Again, the absence of adjustment for confounders and covariates is a biased estimate of the effect. This is an error we should address in the analysis.

Multivariable regression analyses also facilitate tests for effect modification or interaction. Effect modification is present when the strength, direction, and/or statistical significance of the relationship between exposure and outcome differ across categories of a third variable. For a general example, say the effect of drug X on tumor size is much stronger for women than for men. This modification or interaction between exposure and gender can be modeled in the regression equation. Consider the following linear regression equation:

$$\hat{Y} = b_0 + b_1 X_1 + b_2 X_2 + b_3 X_3 + b_4 X_4 + b_5 X_3 * X_4$$

This equation shows two different tests concerning the effects of independent variables on $\hat{Y}$. Like simple regression, b_1 indicates the effect of X_1 on $\hat{Y}$. However, with the inclusion of other Xs in the model, the coefficient for X_1 is adjusted for the effects of the other variables. The coefficient is the effect of X_1 while X_2, X_3, and X_4 are "held constant" or are not permitted to vary.

Effect modification is also tested in this regression model. The effect modification is represented by an interaction term. In this example, we are testing for an interaction between X_3 and X_4. The interaction term multiplies the two variables, and the coefficient b_5 indicates the interactive effect of X_3 and X_4 on $\hat{Y}$. If b_5 is statistically significant, then interaction is present. The R-square for the multivariable model indicates the percent of variation in $\hat{Y}$ that is explained by all of the Xs in the model.

Multivariable models can be tested using many of the statistical procedures we have already covered. These include all of the regression methods (linear, logistic, and Cox proportional hazards) and factorial ANOVA (ANOVA with more than one independent variable). No matter what procedure is used, care must be taken in setting up the models. Prior to testing the model, the coding and recoding of all variables should be correct and make conceptual sense. Continuous measures should be coded in a meaningful direction (i.e., highest to lowest, lowest to highest), dummy variables should be created for dichotomous predictors and the coefficient interpreted properly (i.e., the effect on $\hat{Y}$ when moving from 0 to 1 on the dummy), and missing data should be addressed appropriately (i.e., imputed or coded as missing). All potential confounders and interactions should be tested. However, there is a limit in terms of statistical power in the number of predictors that can be included in models with small samples.

INTERPRETING THE RESULTS (APPROPRIATELY)

We are done! The data are analyzed, and the research question is answered. So, we are done, right? Wrong, of course, because we are reading another section of this chapter. We have one more chance to make a mistake and introduce bias in our study. We can make a conclusion bias. Yes, there really is such a thing, and it is often overlooked because we are exhausted and elated that we have designed the study, reviewed the literature, created the measures, selected the sample, collected the data, and analyzed the results. After all that work, we do not want to waste it by presenting and interpreting the results inappropriately. The guideposts for avoiding conclusion bias are probably best communicated in a "do and don't" list.

- ***Don't*** *attempt the impossible.* If your study is not designed to answer a particular research question, don't even try. A causal question cannot be addressed in cross-sectional study. The causes of depression cannot be examined using an outcome measuring general and vague sadness. Whatever answer you find when you attempt the impossible will be biased.

- ***Do*** *study up on the method(s) you will be using in your analysis.* Learn the procedures, requirement, and assumptions for candidate methods, and make an informed choice. Make sure you have the knowledge to perform the procedure correctly. Be sure you really know what the results mean.

- ***Don't*** *go fishing.* This is the phrase used for analysis that looks at most or all possible relationships until significant ones are found. Odds are you will find a significant relationship if you look at enough of them. Many or most of these "fished for" significant relationships probably make little conceptual sense. They are not worth reporting.

- ***Do*** *double check your assumptions.* Are the residual errors *really* normally distributed? Are the events of death and dropping out of the study really independent? Do you really have enough power to test that many predictor variables in one model? Do you have too many 0 cells? Results of procedures with violated assumptions are biased.

- ***Don't*** *sweep the dirt under the rug.* If the relationship you expected to find is not statistically significant, don't ignore it. Report and speculate why it is not significant. If there is good reason to think gender might be a confounder, test it and report it. Recall that unrecognized confounding is a type of bias. If one of your measures of interest has tons of missing data, don't analyze it as if everything is fine.

- ***Do*** *modify your research plan if you must.* Very little ever occurs exactly as we anticipate. Measures may not work as we planned. There may be only 5% smokers in our study of smoking behavior. We have invested too much to walk away from the data. We need to be creative to cull the best possible analysis out of the data we get. Scale down the scope. Go in a slightly different direction.

- ***Don't*** *reach too high.* Generalizing too broadly is a relatively common mistake. Don't generalize to a target population if you have a biased sample. Don't generalize to the entire U.S. population if your target population is Kansas. Don't interpret or discuss results that you don't have. If you didn't measure self-esteem, don't discuss its role in a relationship. Every conclusion must be supported by meaningful results.

- **Do** *distinguish between types of significance.* Interpret the results in terms of statistical and conceptual/clinical significance. If it is not conceptually significant, it is not important no matter how low the *p*-value. On the other hand, a strong and conceptually meaningful result may not be statistically significant if the study has inadequate power. Perhaps the critical *p*-value should be raised to 0.10. If it is meaningful and strong enough, the relationship should be discussed with caveats about its statistical significance.

- **Don't** *"fudge" the data.* This term refers to manipulating the data until a desired result is found. It is appropriate to "tweak" the data to make the most powerful and correct recode, to analyze the appropriate subset of the data, and so on. But tweaking becomes fudging when the manipulations are extensive, not particularly meaningful, and the only way that significant results can be found.

- **Do** *think about scale.* As discussed earlier in this chapter, choose a scale that reflects the true meaning of a relationship. If the relationship is conceptually weak, don't focus the scale so much that it looks bigger than it is.

- **Don't** *miss the forest for the trees.* If you find a result that does not fit into or reflect the big picture of your research, don't inflate its importance by giving it too much focus. Remind yourself of the broad landscape of your research question.

- **Do** *consult an expert.* It can take years to master even a handful of statistical procedures. We learn a lot by trial and error. If you are new to research or a particular procedure, show your results to an experienced professor or colleague to make sure you are not making the mistakes addressed in this section of the chapter.

CONCLUSION

We just skimmed the surface of statistical methods in this chapter. The reader is encouraged to use the information in this chapter to choose the appropriate family of methods and to avoid introducing bias in the analysis and interpretation of results. There are so many different study designs and research questions that it is impossible to cover all the relevant details in one chapter or even one book. For most methods and types of studies, there is a broad array of published information available for the reader to consult. The first and probably most important step is to choose the correct family of analytic procedures given the study focus and design. With the correct choice, relevant details are fairly easy to locate.

The most important focus of this chapter is to avoid using the wrong methods and reporting biased results. Statistics can be powerful persuaders, sometimes even the difference between life and death. Decision makers who use statistics but may not be the most informed consumers can make policy or design programs or use drug X based on weak or incorrect results. The consequence is a waste of money and time and, at the extreme, harm from missed opportunities or wrong approaches.

A final note about bias in research results should go without saying, but it must be said. It is wrong to falsify data, which ranges from "fudging" to outright fabrication. There is often tremendous pressure to "find results," often when there are inadequate resources. From a publishing standpoint, there is pressure to find significant results. In fact, publication biases results from the fact that statistically significant results are more likely to be published than nonsignificant results, even if they are not particularly meaningful clinically or conceptually. The pressure to produce and publish and get funding should never compromise research integrity in any way, especially in public health research where people's lives could be at stake.

VOCABULARY

Analysis of variance	Intercept	Risk difference
Box-Whisker plot	Interquartile range	Risk ratio
Categorical	Kaplan-Meier	R-square
Confidence interval	Mean	Scales
Continuous	Median	Slope
Chi-square	Missing data	Standard deviation
Cochran-Mantel-	Mode	Statistical significance
Haenszel	Odds ratio	Survival analysis
Correlation	Ordinal	t-score
Crosstab	Pearson correlation	Variable
Descriptive	coefficient	Variance
Dichotomous	Publication bias	Z-score
Dummy variable	p-value	
F-statistic	Range	
Hazard ratio	Raw data	
Imputation	Recode	

STUDY QUESTIONS AND EXERCISES

1. List and describe the appropriate descriptive analysis strategies for the following outcome measures:
   a. Pain is changed or unchanged.
   b. Pain is measured as absent, modest, or severe.
   c. Pain is measured on a 10-point scale where 0 is no pain and 10 is unbearable pain.

2. List and describe the appropriate inferential analysis strategies for each of the outcome measures listed in problem 1.

3. Fix the variables in the table below in order to make their relationship analyzable.

Number of Times Residents Exercise per Week

City residence	None	1–2	3–4	5+	TOTAL
Center	30	105	10	5	150
Fringe	15	100	5	5	125
Near suburbs	25	45	30	0	100
Far suburbs	20	30	25	0	75
Rural	10	20	5	15	50
TOTAL	100	300	75	25	500

4. Create a hypothetical scale measuring health status. Include a full description of each component in the scale as well as how it is measured. Indicate how the components will be combined to create the scale.

5. Draft a brief analysis plan to address each of the following research questions:
   a. What are the health effects of hydraulic fracturing to obtain natural gas?
   b. Do cholesterol-lowering medications cause muscle disorders?
   c. How long can a patient live following a diagnosis of pancreatic cancer?

6. Define and give an example of each of the following types of analysis bias:
   a. Confounding
   b. Conclusion bias
   c. Publication bias

7. Draft the analysis plan for your own study. Include information about:
   a. Descriptive analyses
   b. Inferential analyses
   c. Empty table shells indicating relationships to be evaluated

REFERENCES

Allison, P. (1995). *Survival analysis using the SAS system.* Cary, NC: SAS Institute.

Best, J. (2001). *Damned lies and statistics: Untangling numbers from the media, politicians, and activists.* Berkeley, CA: University of California Press.

Bush, H. M. (2012). *Biostatistics: An applied introduction for the public health practitioner* (1st ed.). Clifton Park, NY: Delmar Cengage Learning.

Chang, M. (2011). *Modern issues and methods in biostatistics.* New York: Springer.

Cox, D. R., & Oakes, D. (1984). *Analysis of survival data.* Boca Raton, FL: Chapman and Hall.

Diggle, P., & Chetwynd, A. (2011). *Statistics and scientific method: An introduction for students and researchers.* New York: Oxford University Press.

Gerstman, B. B. (2008). *Basic biostatistics: Statistics for public health practice.* Sudbury, MA: Jones and Bartlett Publishers.

Glantz, S. A. (2011). *Primer of biostatistics* (7th ed.). New York: McGraw-Hill.

Hebel, J. R., & McCarter, R. J. (2012). *A study guide to epidemiology and biostatistics* (7th wed.). Sudbury, MA: Jones & Bartlett Learning.

Holmes, T. H., & Rahe, R. H. (1967). The social readjustment rating scale. *Journal of Psychosomatic Research, 11*(2), 213–218.

Källén, A. (2011). *Understanding biostatistics.* Chichester, West Sussex, United Kingdom: John Wiley & Sons.

Katz, M. H. (2011). *Multivariable analysis: A practical guide for clinicians and public health researchers* (3rd ed.). Cambridge, NY: Cambridge University Press.

Kleinbaum, D. G., & Klein, M. (2005). *Survival analysis: A self-learning text.* New York: Springer Science + Business Media.

Lachin, J. M. (2011). *Biostatistical methods: The assessment of relative risks* (2nd ed.). Hoboken, NJ: Wiley.

Lee, E. T., & Wang, J. W. (2003). *Statistical methods for survival data analysis* (3rd ed.). New York: John Wiley & Sons.

Merrill, R. M. (2013). *Fundamentals of epidemiology and biostatistics: Combining the basics.* Burlington, MA: Jones & Bartlett Learning.

Rossi, R. J. (2010). *Applied biostatistics for the health sciences.* Hoboken, NJ: John Wiley & Sons.

SAS. (2002–2003). (Version 9.1 ed.). Cary, NC: SAS Institute.

Selvin, S. (2008). *Survival analysis for epidemiologic and medical research: A practical guide.* New York: Cambridge University Press.

Sullivan, L. M. (2012). *Essentials of biostatistics in public health* (2nd ed.). Sudbury, MA: Jones & Bartlett Learning.

Vittinghoff, E. (2011). *Regression methods in biostatistics: Linear, logistic, survival, and repeated measures models.* New York: Springer.

CHAPTER 10

Interpreting Results

LEARNING OBJECTIVES

By the end of this chapter the reader will be able to:
- Interpret the results of basic computer printout correctly.
- Translate computer printout into reportable results.
- Address unanticipated results.
- Interpret study results correctly.
- Interpret study results ethically.

CHAPTER OUTLINE

There are three kinds of lies: lies, damned lies, and statistics.
  —Benjamin Disraeli or maybe Eliza Gutch or
    maybe Walter Bagehot or maybe Arthur James
    Balfour or maybe Leonard H. Courtney or maybe …?

INTRODUCTION

Even though we do not know who said it for certain, this popular quotation highlights the danger of misinterpreting statistics or study results either by mistake or as part of a predetermined agenda. This process of "lying" is complicated because it can come from many sources: lying by design, by omission, or by naiveté. No matter the source, it is truly unethical, misleading, and perhaps harmful to interpret study results inaccurately. Findings adapted by policy makers and program planners may not be appropriately vetted depending on the expertise of the makers and planners. It is the responsibility of the researcher to interpret the results in a way that makes them useful as accurate "evidence" in evidence-based programming.

There are multitudes of research questions, hypotheses, study designs, types of data, and analytic techniques that fit under the umbrella of public health research. Of course, it is impossible to address the issues of interpretation for all of these potential studies, but it is important for the reader to get a concrete idea of the issues involved in the interpretation of results. Therefore, we will work through a specific, rather simple study that represents some of the issues likely to be confronted by the novice researcher, and we will interpret an example SAS printout (SAS, 2002–2003).

CONFRONTING A BUNCH OF NUMBERS

Look at **Figures 10–1 to 10–3**. We are confronting a bunch of numbers. We will address each number in turn—what it means both statistically and conceptually. Through this process, we will examine the appropriate statistics and decide which we should report in relationship to our hypothesis or research question. We will not pick and choose statistics that only support our hypothesis. We will report what is relevant and unique. But first, let us put the numbers in context.

Say for your thesis, you have chosen to examine the potential association between subjects' parents' health history and subjects' own general health status. The hypothesis is that there is a positive relationship between parents' health history and subjects' health status. You use a cross-sectional survey data set with 100 adult subjects from a mid-sized Midwest city and 50 variables about health status, parents' health history, health-related behaviors, and demographic characteristics. The main component of your analysis is the examination of the association between the independent variable (parents' health history measured as an additive scale combining all negative health events and risk behaviors, such as cigarette smoking, diabetes, heart disease, etc.) and the dependent variable (subjects' own health status measured as an additive scale combining relevant negative health measures, such as heavy alcohol use, high blood pressure, high

Moments			
N	100	Sum Weights	100
Mean	52.775	Sum Observations	5278
Std Deviation	18.9571720	Variance	179.687180
Skewness	-0.4820386	Kurtosis	-0.7502476
Uncorrected SS	574919	Corrected SS	17878.875
Coeff Variation	17.9603714	Std Error Mean	1.3404744

Basic Statistical Measures			
Location		Variability	
Mean	52.77500	Std Deviation	18.95717
Median	54.00000	Variance	179.69718
Mode	59.00000	Range	36.00000
		Interquartile Range	14.50000

FIGURE 10–1 Example SAS Output of Basic Descriptive Statistics (The Univariate Procedure)

The CORR Procedure

3 Variables: risk health female
Simple Statistics

Variable	Label	N	Mean	Std Dev	Sum	Minimum	Maximum
Risk	Family risk score	100	52.23000	20.50588	5278	28.00000	76.00000
Health	Health score	100	52.77500	18.95717	5226	31.00000	67.00000
Female		100	0.54500	0.49922	59.00000	0	1.00000

Pearson Correlation Coefficients, $N = 100$
Prob > |r| under $H0$: $Rho = 0$

	Risk	Health	Female
Risk	1.00000	0.0628	-0.05308
Family risk score		0.3889	0.4553
Health	0.0628	1.00000	-0.25649
Health score	0.3889		0.0273
Female	-0.05308	-0.25649	1.00000
	0.4553	0.0273	

FIGURE 10–2 Example SAS Output of the Correlation Between Three Variables (Correlation Procedure)

Dependent Variable: Health Score

Analysis of Variance

Source		DF	Sum of Squares	Mean Square	F Value	Pr > F
Model		2	318.43003	159.21500	3.10	< .05
Error		97	4981.88963	51.35968		
Corrected total		99	5300			
Root MSE		7.16656	R-Square	0.1896		
Dependent mean		51.85000	Adj R-Sq	0.1734		
Coeff var		13.82171				

Parameter Estimates

Variable	Label	DF	Parameter Estimate	Standard Error	t Value	Pr > |t|
Intercept	Intercept	1	12.32529	3.19356	3.86	0.0002
Risk	Parent risk score	1	0.19465	0.28645	1.12	0.3061
Female		1	−2.69998	1.02272	−2.64	0.0098

Parameter Estimates

Variable	Label	DF	95% Confidence	Limits
Intercept	Intercept	1	0.32529	24.32529
Risk	Parent risk score	1	−0.48111	0.91800
Female		1	−1.67708	−3.72252

FIGURE 10–3 Example SAS Output of Multiple Linear Regression (Regression Procedure)

total cholesterol, high blood sugar, etc.). The higher the values on both scale measures of parents' and own health, the worse the health status. You also plan to examine subjects' gender as a potential confounder in the relationship between parents' health history and subjects' health status. The typical thesis would have a more comprehensive analysis plan, but we will focus on this portion of the analysis as an example.

You first examine both scale measures to determine their important characteristics, such as missing data and descriptive statistics. Results of the SAS univariate procedure ("proc univariate") analyzing the dependent variable (health status) are presented in Figure 10–1. We will discuss each component of the output. First, "Moments" are descriptive statistics of the distribution of the dependent variable called HEALTH. N is the number of valid responses for the variable HEALTH. The N value is 100, so we know that we do not have any missing data. The mean or arithmetic average of the scale is 52.78, and the standard deviation measure of dispersion is 18.96. We will talk more about these shortly. Skewness measures the degree and direction of asymmetry of the distribution of HEALTH. A symmetric distribution is a normal distribution. The value of skewness for a normal distribution is zero (0). Therefore, the larger the value, the greater is the degree of skewness. A positive value indicates positive skewness (i.e., outliers on the high end of the distribution), and a negative value indicates the existence of outliers on the lower end. The skewness value for HEALTH is −0.48, so the distribution is relatively symmetrical (i.e., the value is close to 0), with limited outliers on the lower end of the distribution. In other words, the sample is somewhat more healthy (with lower values on the scale) than unhealthy. Because the degree of skewness is relatively minor, it is appropriate to use procedures dependent on the mean rather than the median as the measure of centrality.

The uncorrected SS is the sum of squared data values, which is a component of the formula for variance and standard deviation. The coefficient of variance—the ratio of the standard deviation (18.96) to the mean (52.78) expressed as a percentage—is 17.96%. A higher percentage indicates a greater relative variation around the mean. This statistic is helpful for comparing standard deviations across different variables, with unique means. It is a form of standardization. The sum of weights indicates the total value for weights assigned to variables to adjust for situations such as over- and under-sampling so that the variable to be analyzed represents the distribution in the sample population. Weights are multiplied by observed data values. Our data is not weighted, so each case is multiplied by one (1) to preserve the original value.

The sum of observations is simply the total of all 100 scale values on the HEALTH variable. Variance is another measure of variation of data around the mean. Kurtosis is another measure of the symmetry of the distribution for HEALTH. The measure compares the height of the distribution tails for HEALTH to those of a hypothetical normal distribution, which has a kurtosis value of zero (0). If kurtosis is positive, the observed tails are heavier (i.e., contain more observations, more extreme values) than those of a normal distribution. If the statistic is negative, the observed tails are lighter (i.e., most of the data clusters closely around the mean or center of the distribution). The kurtosis value for HEALTH is −0.75, is close to 0, and indicates that the observed data cluster closely around the mean. Again, this value supports the use of methods based on the mean for the HEALTH variable. The corrected SS is the sum of the squared deviations around the mean. This measure is used to calculate the variance and standard deviation. (Note: The uncorrected SS is the sum of the squared data values, without consideration of their distance from the mean.) The standard error of the mean is the sample standard deviation divided by the square root of N. This is the value we would expect if we drew 100 samples and calculated the mean for each and then calculated the standard deviation of the 100 means around the overall mean for the distribution of 100 means. This is a measure of variability of the population mean.

The mean, median, and mode are the three measures of centrality. The median is not sensitive to outliers and is the value that separates the lower and higher halves of the distribution. A comparison of the values of the mean and median further shows that the distribution of HEALTH is slightly negatively skewed. The mean value is smaller than the median because the mean is being pulled to the left by extreme values on the lower end of the distribution. The range is the difference between the highest and lowest values on the distribution of HEALTH. The interquartile range is the difference between the value separating the lower 75% of the distribution and the value separating the lower 25% of the distribution.

The next step in the analysis would be to examine the bivariable relationships between HEALTH and the other variables of interest. Because HEALTH is a continuous measure, we can use Pearson's correlation coefficients in the SAS correlation procedure (PROC CORR). Sample output of the correlation analysis is shown in Figure 10–2. The correlation procedure presents the descriptive statistics for each variable included in the correlation analysis. Moments for RISK from parents' health and GENDER (and any other variables included in the overall analysis) should be reported. Methods for choosing the appropriate statistics to report will be discussed in the next section. In addition, it is informative to report the minimum and maximum values of each variable to help put the mean, standard deviation, and range in the context of scale. The minimum and maximum values of 31.0 and 67.0 for the health status measure can be added to **Table 10–1** to show the end values for the range of 36.0. Descriptive labels for variables (beyond the sometimes vague one-word variable name) are also provided if the labels were created at data entry or variable transformation. The measure of gender is a dummy variable with male coded as "0" and female coded as "1." As a dummy variable, the dichotomous measure can be treated

Table 10–1 Example Presentation of Descriptive Statistics

Variable	N	Mean (std. dev.)	Minimum–maximum values	Skewness
Health status	100	52.8 (19.0)	31.0–67.0	−0.5
Family risk	100	52.2 (20.5)	28.0–76.0	—
Female	100	0.54 (—)	0–1	—

— Data not presented
Note: The measure for gender (female) is coded "0" for males and "1" for females.

like a continuous measure, with a regression coefficient showing the change in $\hat{Y}$ comparing females to males. Hence, the dummy variable is called FEMALE.

Pearson correlation coefficients (r) for the three variables included in the analysis (independent, dependent, and potential confounder) are presented in matrix form. Each variable has a row and a column in the matrix. The matrix shows the correlations between all possible pairs of variables, including each variable correlated with itself, which will always be 1.0. Values listed just under each coefficient are the probability values from tests of statistical significance. The hypothesis that r is not equal to 0.0 is tested. If p is less than or equal to 0.05, the correlation coefficient is considered to be statistically significant, significantly different than 0.0.

Considering the correlation between each pair of variables, the matrix shows that the correlation between family risk (independent variable) and health status (dependent variable) is 0.06, with a p-value of 0.3889. The correlation between gender (potential confounder) and health status (dependent variable) is −0.26 ($p = 0.0273$) and between gender (potential confounder) and family risk (independent variables) is −0.05 ($p = 0.4552$). We will discuss these results a little later.

The last step in this small portion of analysis for the thesis is multiple regression analysis with which we can examine the change in health status from changes in family risk and gender simultaneously. For this step, we use the regression procedure (PROC REG) in SAS. The printout is presented in Figure 10–3. The first portion of the printout shows results of the analysis of variance (ANOVA) comparing the mean values of health status for the subgroups defined by family risk and gender. Source refers to the source of variance in health status. Model source is the variance in health status explained by family risk and gender. Error source is the remaining variation not explained by the two variables in the model. Corrected total source is a combination of model and error variance. Each source of variance has its own degree of freedom (df). The model source df is the number of parameters to be estimated in the regression equation (intercept, slope for family risk, and slope for gender or 3 parameters) minus 1 (model $df = 3 - 1$, or 2). The degrees of freedom for the error source are the remaining degrees of freedom or N minus the number of parameters to be estimated ($df = 100 - 3$, or 97). The total degrees of freedom are the sum of the model and error degrees of freedom ($2 + 97 = 99$).

The sum of squares is the sum of the squared deviation from the mean of health status for the model, the error, and the total. The mean square values are the sum of squares divided by their respective degrees of freedom. The mean for the model source sum of squares, for example, is $318.43003/2 = 159.21500$.

This value and the mean square for the error source are used to calculate the F statistic—the test statistic to determine statistical significance for ANOVA ($F = \text{MSM/MSE}$). In this example, the F value of 3.10 ($= 159.21500/51.35968$) is statistically significant ($p < 0.05$) for $df = 2$ and 97. Based on these results, we can reject the null hypothesis that the means of health status are equal across subgroups defined by parent risk and gender, or that the estimated parameters are all equal to 0.

The remaining statistics in the ANOVA section of the printout indicate the degree of overall fit of the model (family risk and gender). Root MSE is the standard deviation of the error source or the square root of the mean square error. The dependent mean is the mean of the dependent variable or the mean of health status. The coefficient of variation is the root MSE divided by the dependent mean and multiplied by 100. This is a standardized measure, expressed as a percentage, indicating the general variation in the data. The R-square value is the proportion of the variance in the dependent variable explained by the variables in the model. This is an overall measure of the strength of association between health status and the combination of family risk and gender. It is sometimes expressed as a percentage, so in our example, family risk and gender explain 19% of the variation in health status. The adjusted R-square accounts for the inclusion of more than one independent measure.

The "parameter estimates" section of the output presents the intercept and slope estimates for the regression equation predicting values of the health status measure. Each parameter has 1 degree of freedom associated with it. According to these estimates, the equation is:

$$\hat{Y} = 12.32 + 0.19 \text{ Parent Risk} - 2.70 \text{ Female}$$

The intercept, or 12.32, is the point on the health risk measure where the regression line begins. The equation facilitates the prediction of health risk based on knowledge of a subject's values on parent risk and gender. For example, a female subject with a parent risk score of 42 would be expected to have a health status score of:

$$12.23 + 0.19 \ (42) - 2.70 \ (1) = 17.51$$

The standard error for each parameter estimate is used to test the statistical significance of each estimate (tested with the t test statistic) and to calculate the confidence intervals. The probability value for each t statistic indicates if the parameter is significantly different than 0. Usually a probability less than or equal to 0.05 is considered statistically significant. Similarly, confidence intervals that do not include the value of 0 indicate that the parameter is significantly different than 0.

PICKING AND CHOOSING (APPROPRIATELY)

So, now, what would we report? What would we conclude? Of course, we want to "describe" our dependent variable (and really all the variables in our analysis) in terms of centrality, variation, size, range, and distribution shape. A table similar to Table 10–1 would be appropriate. We would interpret these statistics by saying, for example:

> The dependent measure of health status is an additive scale of X items measuring health problems, including higher than normal total cholesterol, blood sugar, blood pressure, and so on. The range of scale values is 36.0 units (maximum of 67.0 minus minimum of 31.0). The mean is 52.8, with a standard deviation of 19.0. A skewness of −0.5 indicates a limited number of extreme values on the lower end of the scale. The health status scale is mildly skewed toward a favorable health status. However, the degree of asymmetry does not preclude the use of analytic methods, namely linear regression analysis, that are based on statistics calculated using the mean of the variable.

We would summarize the statistics for the other two variables in the analysis in a similar fashion. The skewness is not reported for family risk because the concern for distribution symmetry is mainly relevant for the dependent variable. This decision is based somewhat on personal preference. Reporting the skewness for independent variables would not be incorrect. The skewness measure for gender, on the other hand, is not meaningful because the measure is a dummy variable with two categories. In addition, the mean for gender is interpreted as the proportion of females in the sample, because females are coded "1" in the dummy variable. Hence, the sample is 54% female. The standard deviation for the dichotomous variable is not reported because it is not meaningful for measures other than continuous.

Moving on to the correlation analysis, the key pieces of data to present are the Pearson correlation coefficient and associated probability value for each pair of variables. **Table 10–2** shows the basic style of presentation of the data. At this point, you as the thesis researcher are likely alarmed, panicked, and perhaps despairing. The correlation between family risk and health status is weak (0.06) and not statistically significant! This is the cornerstone of your analysis! Take a

Table 10–2 Example Presentation of Pearson Correlation Coefficients

Variable	Health status	Family risk	Female
Health status	1.00	0.06	−0.26*
Family risk		1.00	−0.05
Female			1.00

*$p < 0.05$
Note: The measure for gender (female) is coded "0" for males and "1" for females.

deep breath. You do not have to scrap the analysis. We will discuss research options in the next section, but for now we would conclude with something like this:

> The correlation coefficient for the relationship between family risk and health status is in the expected direction (i.e., the greater the risk, the worse the health status), but the magnitude is weak and is not statistically significant. The magnitude is so weak that the lack of statistical significance is likely not due to a lack of statistical power with a sample size of 100. [We will explore this relationship in more detail shortly.] The coefficient for the relationship between female and family risk is also weak and not significant, but the correlation between female gender and health status is moderate in strength and statistically significant ($r = -0.26$; $p < 0.05$). The negative direction of the coefficient indicates that females compared to males have an overall better health status.

The last component of this portion of the analysis is the multivariable test of the relationships between family risk and health, and female gender and health. The SAS output for the regression procedure (PROC REG) is shown in Figure 10–3.

The relevant statistics from the regression procedure are the adjusted R-square, the regression coefficients, and the statistical significance. Depending on the discipline and journal or academic requirements, the probability values or the confidence intervals should be presented to show statistical significance. Both can be and sometimes are presented, but it is sometimes a matter of opinion as to the need to present both. Similarly, for the purposes of this example, there is no need to present the ANOVA results in full. What is useful to add to the regression results is the fact that the Model F statistic is statistically significant, which indicates that health status means are significantly different between subgroups defined by family risk and gender. The R-square is a more meaningful indicator of the overall association between the model (all independent variables) and the outcome, but no test of statistical significance is available for the R-square. Results of the F test add that piece of information. Example results are presented in **Table 10–3**.

As expected from the results of the correlation procedure, family risk does not have a statistically significant effect on health status. However, gender still has a

Table 10–3 Example Presentation of Multiple Regression Results

	Parameter	(95% CI)	Adj. R-Square	F-Statistic
Intercept	12.32	(0.32, 24.32)		
Family risk	0.19	(−0.48, 0.92)		
Female	−2.70	(−3.72, −1.68)		
MODEL			0.17	3.10*

*$p < 0.05$
Note: The measure for gender (female) is coded "0" for males and "1" for females.

significant effect on health status even when controlling for family risk. These results would be summarized similar to the following:

> Results of the regression analysis indicate that family risk does not have a significant effect on health status. On the other hand, gender (female) has a negative statistically significant effect ($p < 0.05$), meaning that females have a lower health status score (really a more favorable status) compared to males. Females have a health score almost 3 units lower than males. The adjusted R-square shows that the three parameters (intercept and both coefficients) account for 17% of the variance in subjects' health status. The F statistic for the ANOVA model indicates that the means of health status for subgroups defined by family risk and gender are significantly different from each other.

ADJUSTING EXPECTATIONS

So, now what? The hypothesis of this portion of your thesis was not supported. We should explore the lack of statistical significance in the relationship between parent risk and health status in greater detail. First, could there be a lack of statistical power? Our sample has an N of 100 with no missing data in the analysis. This sample size should be sufficient to detect a two-way correlation between two continuous measures with relatively symmetrical distributions. In other words, there should be very few if any cells in the two-way table with values of zero (0). Such empty cells limit the ability to detect statistical significance. This should not be a problem.

The direction of the correlation coefficient is in the expected direction—the greater the family risk, the more adverse the health status. However, the magnitude is extremely weak ($r = 0.06$). This weak relationship suggests that the lack of statistical significance in the correlation is likely a "real" finding. Family risk is not associated with subjects' health status. Does this mean that a person's health is not related to her parents' health? Genetics and family environment make no difference in one's health? Not likely, based on the results of decades of epidemiologic research.

So, now what? Perhaps, we do not have a valid measure of family risk (or even of health status). One way to begin examining the validity of these measures is an exploration of predictive validity. Are the measures associated with other measures that, intuitively and based on previous research, they should be? Your data set has some variables that can be examined for this purpose. You correlate the parents' age of death (premature or not) with the family risk measure and find a weak relationship that is not statistically significant. The age of death variable has very little missing data (say, three cases) and an acceptable distribution (25% premature), so the lack of significance is likely a "real" result. This (lack of) result leads you to doubt the validity of your family risk measure. Additional relevant analysis would examine correlations between matched components of the family risk and health status scales to the extent possible given the distributions of each component. You find that the parents' diabetes is associated with the subjects' diabetes. The parents' and subjects' obesity is correlated. However, most of the behavioral risk factors (cigarette smoking, high-fat diet, excessive alcohol use, etc.) are not correlated. Perhaps the family risk scale is a valid measure of genetic predisposition, but its relationship with subject health status is diluted by differences in risk behaviors between subjects and their parents. But you still proceed with caution because family risk should be related to the parents' premature death. You should examine as many correlations as possible between family risk and other potential predictive validity measures to try to accurately characterize the concept that this scale actually measures. It may be appropriate to create subscales using related subgroups of variables in the family risk scale (e.g., health risk behaviors, likely inherited disorders) and use these in analyses with subjects' health status.

So, now what? Actually, this separation of risk behavior and inherited conditions could be an interesting difference to examine further. Are subjects less likely to engage in health-risk behaviors if their parents did? If so, does this difference act as a protector for subjects' health status? These questions can be answered by examining the correlations between the parents' and subjects' individual health behaviors. If some or most are statistically significant and negative in direction (i.e., the parents' smoking is related to the subjects' not smoking), then you may be onto something. Your research question can now be adjusted to examine the differential effects of the parents' disorders and risk behaviors on the subjects' health status. It is very important to note that this adjustment is NOT the result of a fishing trip through the data. You did not look at most or all potential correlations in your data and then zero in on the ones that are statistically significant. You began with and tested a reasonable hypothesis—one based on previous strong research. The lack of association between family risk and health status is unexpected. Your investigation to determine why there is no significant relationship led you to other related research questions and hypotheses. This is real-world (not textbook) research.

So, now what else? You still do have a significant correlation between gender and health status. This was not the centerpiece of your study, but a portion of your analysis can explore this relationship further. You can examine gender differences in health risk behaviors and differences in health problems. Perhaps there are other relevant measures in the data set that make sense to compare by gender. This expansion of gender relationships is justified by the initial inclusion of gender as a potential confounder in this portion of your analysis.

ANSWERING THE RESEARCH QUESTION(S)

Is there a relationship between the parents' health problems and the subjects' health status? As is often the case, your results support the answer "yes and no." Like many relationships in epidemiology, this one is complex. Your results suggest that the family risk measure is multidimensional. On a general level, there are two dimensions: manifestation of inherited factors (e.g., parent and subject diabetes), and behavioral factors (e.g., heavy alcohol use). However, these two dimensions often work together to influence health—a parent with diabetes is also obese. With 100 subjects and self-reported data, your study can go only so far to tease out the complexity of these dimensions and relationships. At this point, you should go back to the literature and search and cite studies (if any) that address the multidimensional aspect of family health risk. The good news is that your results suggest specific directions for future research. You have made a contribution to the scientific method.

This brings us to the treatment of the potential or real limitations of your study. The important focus is on sources of bias that may affect the relationship between family risk and the subjects' own health status. Such limitations may also play a role in the fact that you did not find a statistically significant relationship between these two measures. Starting with the broader picture, do you have sufficient external or even internal validity? Is your sample representative of the intended target population? Do you have selection or nonresponse bias? If you collected your own data, you have already addressed this in the conduct of your study. If this is a secondary analysis of existing data, you will need to review the documentation of data collection and note the limitations acknowledged by the original investigators. You should also evaluate the sampling frame and procedures yourself to make sure there are not limitations that may affect your research question specifically, or that may have been overlooked by the original investigators. A sample size of 100 subjects chosen from a complete and accurate sampling frame using the best possible probability sampling method with at least an 80% response rate should be sufficient for this level of analysis. Your job is to try to evaluate the sampling frame, sampling technique, and response rate. If you see or suspect selection or nonresponse bias, you could speculate that you may have found a significant relationship among individuals that were not included in the study. It would be insightful to compare your sample characteristics to those of studies that did find a significant relationship to speculate about potential sources of bias in your sample.

Another area of potential bias is in the measurement of family risk and health status. Ideally, these concepts would be measured as objectively as possible and even verified with alternative sources. For example, medical records of both parents and subjects would be reviewed to help evaluate the validity of subjects' self-reports. Self-reports have the potential for significant measurement bias, but they are often the most practical methods of measurement. Potential measurement problems can be the results of recall bias and simply a lack of knowledge about the parents' and even the subjects' own health status. Health problems could be forgotten, hidden (by parents from children), or undiagnosed.

Threats to content validity are another source of potential bias. Perhaps all of the important dimensions of family risk are not included in the measure, or, as we have already addressed, the different dimensions are related to each other in ways that may deflate the relationship between this measure and health status. There are analytic techniques, such as factor analysis, that can address this issue, at least in part. An examination of the correlation matrix of every pair of the measures included in the family risk scale can also show items that do not fit in the scale (i.e., they are not correlated with any of the other items). On the other hand, pairs that are very highly correlated (e.g., $r > 0.8$) might be measuring essentially the same concept, and only one should be included in the scale. Generally, again, it could be insightful to compare your measures to those of studies that did find a significant relationship to determine potential weaknesses in your measures.

Confounding can also be a problem in cross-sectional studies. In this case, negative confounding, where the crude relationship is weaker than the adjusted relationship, would be the problem. This type of confounding is not the most common type, but this possibility should be addressed to the extent possible and practical. Potential confounders could be tested analytically. The nature of the confounder should make sense. Examining potential confounders without support from previous studies or good conceptual justification is a fishing trip not a scientific inquiry.

Given your study design and types of measurement, these are the most likely sources of bias. The important point here is to spend time thinking about your results. Go back to the studies you examined in your literature review and search for additional studies about results you did not anticipate. Comparisons of your study characteristics (e.g., nature of the sample, types of measures) to others may suggest potential reasons for conflicting or new results. This process links your study to the past and suggests direction for future parts of the scientific method examining the topic of your research.

CONCLUSION

The purpose of this chapter was to work through a specific research question, study design, and analysis to demonstrate methods for reporting and interpreting example results. In the end, researchers are limited by their study results, which are rarely their ideal. Barring extreme and serious failings in the conduct of the study, researchers should strive to make the absolute best of their study results. Problematic results (i.e., somewhat biased or unreliable) are still worth reporting, as long as the problems are addressed as best as possible. Problems are addressed by additional analyses, comparisons to other studies, and educated speculation. Any conclusions drawn from the study should be made in light of carefully evaluated and clearly stated caveats about potential sources of bias in the study. For the researcher reading your research report, the obvious implication from your evaluation of your results would be to use designs and create measures intended to overcome these limitations. For the designer of interventions or the policy maker, you have offered a realistic evaluation of your results so that the designer or policy maker can decide for him- or herself if your research "evidence" is robust enough to use in the practice of promotion and prevention.

The scientific method is the pursuit of "truth." Researchers who make a real contribution to this pursuit are those that strive for maximal validity and who thoughtfully evaluate the threats to validity in the results they report. Such researchers use methods they understand, design studies and analyses that are as robust as possible and practical, focus their analyses on the research question or hypothesis, report results that address the question or hypothesis, and honestly evaluate the validity of their results. Those who stray from these goals, whether intentionally or unintentionally, present results that are untrue and/or misleading. The end result is a detour from the path to truth. This detour is unscientific and unethical. It is the intentional or unintentional misuse of statistics. The detour can be slight, but it is the responsibility of the researcher to recognize and acknowledge the detour and, to the extent possible, get back on the right path.

The primary goal of the novice researcher is to learn about threats to study validity, as well as strategies to overcome them. Books and classes provide some of this education, but even seasoned researchers seek the consultation of colleagues with relevant expertise. This is an important part of the scientific method. Consultations can focus on all aspects of the study, from design to interpretation of results. The student researcher has faculty, mentors, principal investigators, and colleagues to consult. The researcher's early career is not possible without the advice and guidance of those with more experience and more refined expertise. Studies and their results should be reviewed by study leaders, faculty, mentors, and formal reviewers. Truly, "two (or more) heads are better than one" when it comes to the fruitful pursuit of scientific truth.

VOCABULARY

F statistic	Mean squares model	R-square
Kurtosis	Mean squares total	Skewness
Mean squares error	Moments	Sum of squares

REFERENCE

SAS. (2002–2003). (Version 9.1 ed.). Cary, NC: SAS Institute.

CHAPTER 11

Reporting Results

LEARNING OBJECTIVES

By the end of this chapter the reader will be able to:

- Summarize research results.
- Distinguish statements that are and are not supported by the results.
- Draft all sections of a research report.
- Prepare correct citations and references.
- Create meaningful data tables and graphs.
- Write with brevity as the goal.

CHAPTER OUTLINE

IX. Title and Abstract
X. Acknowledgments
XI. CONSORT and STROBE
XII. Conclusion
XIII. Vocabulary

All we need are the facts, ma'am.

—Sergeant Joe Friday, *Dragnet* TV Series, 1951

INTRODUCTION

This may be one of the most parodied (and misquoted) quotations in popular culture. However, its meaning is relevant for the topic of this chapter. When the character Sergeant Friday from the old television series *Dragnet* interviewed crime witnesses, he would try to limit their narrative to information directly relevant to the crime. Research reports should do the same—limit statements to only those supported by research results. Journal space is at a premium, and readers' (including thesis advisers') attention spans are limited. A report that efficiently makes the point with results that support it is a strong report. Reports that make points not supported by results are misleading and probably a waste of the readers' time.

The information presented in this chapter should be treated like a culinary recipe. The novice cook would follow the recipe exactly, because he or she lacks the experience to prepare the dish without guidance. On the other hand, the experienced chef would use the recipe as a guide and make appropriate changes based on the tastes of his or her diners. Some ingredients are indispensible and some procedures necessary, but the recipe as a whole can be modified according to the taste of the cook and the availability of ingredients and equipment. Generally, if the reader follows the recipe presented in this chapter, the end result will be a research report or journal article manuscript that meets most requirements. However, required specific ingredients and procedures will vary by professor/adviser, research institute, and professional journal. Most journals outline these requirements in sections usually called "Information for Authors." The researcher should be clear about the relevant specific requirements before beginning the first draft. An example "Information for Authors" is presented later in this chapter.

The "recipe" presented in this chapter is for a generic manuscript for a journal article or research report. The manuscript should be double-spaced, using 11-point

Times New Roman font for text, and should be about 10 pages long excluding the abstract, acknowledgments, tables, figures, and references. Adequately covering the relevant information within this length or slightly shorter is the ideal. Considerably longer manuscripts may require editing for superfluous information or "wordiness," or considered for separation into two or more manuscripts.

SHAPE OF THE REPORT

The research report can be conceptualized as having a shape in terms of the level of focus. The shape is an hourglass—wide for a broad focus and narrow for a specific focus (Bem, 2004). The focus begins broadly in the introduction, narrows to the results, then broadens again to the conclusion. The shape is illustrated in **Figure 11–1**.

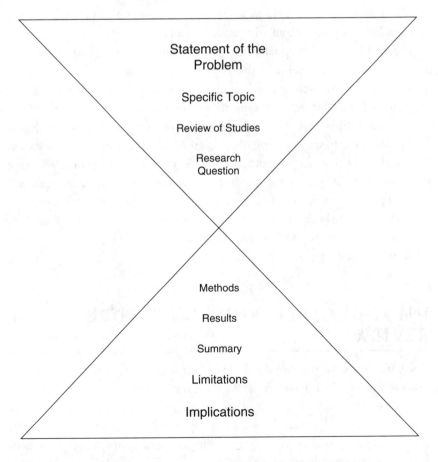

FIGURE 11–1 Hourglass Shape of a Research Report

The significance of the study in terms of its implications for a broader problem or issue is communicated in the first sentence of the report. Next, relevant studies that address the specific aspect of the broader problem are reviewed. From this review, the research question or hypothesis emerges. A description of the specific study design follows. Results are presented. Results are summarized in the context of the research question or hypothesis. Limitations of the study are addressed. Conclusions and implications are drawn. Suggestions for the next step in research on the topic are made.

The review of prior studies and the suggestions for future inquiry represent the scientific method. The method begins with hypotheses or questions generated by prior studies or observations. The hypothesis is tested in the current study, and, ideally, the results stimulate additional hypotheses and research. The report draws from what is known, provides new knowledge, and guides the way to the pursuit of additional knowledge. As a link in the chain of the scientific process, it is vital that our link is strong by being the result of valid inquiry.

Figure 11–2 presents specific examples of statements representing changing levels of focus in the report. In this example report, heart disease is the broad problem being addressed. Previous studies suggest a promising intervention to help prevent heart disease. This study demonstrates its effectiveness, given certain limitations of the sample. The researchers conclude that the intervention should be implemented to prevent heart disease. In addition, the intervention should be tested in other studies without this study's limitations. The hourglass shape of the report is anchored in the middle by the research question: Does a diet and exercise program result in a greater improvement in cholesterol levels compared to each behavior alone, or neither? The introduction of the report rationalizes and concludes with the question, and the discussion section begins with and then answers the question.

INTRODUCTION AND LITERATURE REVIEW

The basic recipe for the introduction has four ingredients. The ingredients are listed in **Figure 11–3**. First is a statement of the importance of the broad issue. In epidemiology, this would be a health-related issue, such as illness, death, disability, or disorder. The introduction begins by identifying the problem and then, briefly, justifying its importance (e.g., leading cause of death, affects millions of people, or costs millions of dollars in work absences). Results from large-scale

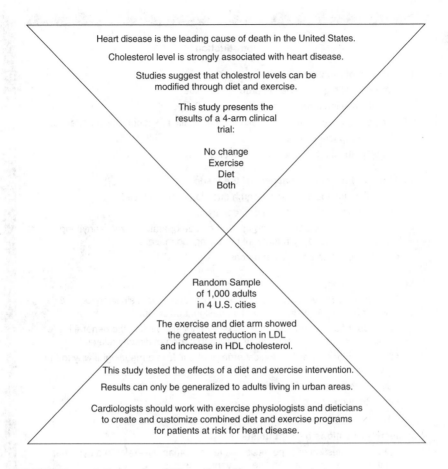

Heart disease is the leading cause of death in the United States.

Cholesterol level is strongly associated with heart disease.

Studies suggest that cholestrol levels can be modified through diet and exercise.

This study presents the results of a 4-arm clinical trial:

No change
Exercise
Diet
Both

Random Sample of 1,000 adults in 4 U.S. cities

The exercise and diet arm showed the greatest reduction in LDL and increase in HDL cholesterol.

This study tested the effects of a diet and exercise intervention.

Results can only be generalized to adults living in urban areas.

Cardiologists should work with exercise physiologists and dieticians to create and customize combined diet and exercise programs for patients at risk for heart disease.

FIGURE 11–2 Example of Hourglass Shape

studies should be reviewed here to support the statement of importance. For our study example, data about leading causes of death can be reviewed. This information can be presented in one paragraph.

Second is a statement of the specific aspect of the broader issue that will be examined in the study. In our example study, the broad issue is heart disease, and the specific focus is ways to improve cholesterol levels and, hopefully, prevent heart disease. This statement introduces the third ingredient—the review of relevant studies. The review should focus exclusively on studies and results that are relevant to the research question. Key characteristics of the studies should be summarized (e.g., target population, procedures), and results should be presented in a manner or order that leads to the presentation of the research question or hypothesis. Brevity and laser focus are important here. If possible, the structure

Introduction

1. **Importance of the broad issue**
   - Introduce the general health problem or issue.
   - Emphasize the magnitude of importance.
   - Review large-scale study or surveillance results to support the importance.
   - Use appropriate citation style.
   - Limit to about a half double-spaced page.

2. **Statement of the specific aspect of the issue**
   - Introduce the focus of the research question or hypothesis.
   - Link the specific focus to the broader issue.
   - Discuss at a level specific enough that can be operationalized—anything broader is misleading in terms of promising too much.
   - Limit to about one or two sentences.

3. **Literature Review**
   - Review only relevant studies—similar target population, similar exposure, similar outcome, similar intervention design, and so on.
   - Limit specificity to the research focus—do not slip back to the general issue or get side-tracked to prior study results that are not directly relevant.
   - Discuss prior studies in a logical order that builds in a meaningful way to the research question.
   - Use appropriate citation style.
   - Limit to about 2 pages.

4. **Research Questions or Hypothesis**
   - State the question or hypothesis in a testable manner—refer to a hypothesis in the context of the alternative relevant to the null.
   - Emphasize that this is the purpose of the present study.
   - Discuss how the test of this research question or hypothesis will extend what is currently known about the specific focus.
   - Limit to about half a page.

FIGURE 11–3 Recipe for the Introduction and Literature Review

of the review should build the results (i.e., from simple to more complex, from oldest to most recent, from broad to specific) in a way to guide the reader to the ultimate conclusion of the research question.

The fourth and final ingredient is the research question or hypothesis. Included with the presentation of the hypothesis is a brief explanation of how this question or hypothesis adds new information beyond the results of the studies reviewed. Perhaps a known exposure is being tested on a different outcome. A new exposure is tested.

A previously demonstrated relationship is examined in a different target population. A modified intervention is evaluated. Ideally, the study contributes to a body of research. It strengthens the proof for causality by replicating a relationship in a different context. Or not . . . results that do not support causality are also important in that they may suggest studies that move in a different direction. Generally, the introduction and literature review should not exceed three double-spaced pages.

METHODS

The ingredients for this section of the report vary somewhat according to the study design. Most generally, the methods section should include a description of the sample, data collection procedures, measures, and analysis procedures. These ingredients are described in **Figure 11–4**. The description should be detailed enough to inform the reader and to allow the reader to evaluate the strength of the study methods. Limitations of the methods can be mentioned here, but their implications should be saved for the discussion section. Generally, all types of implications should be reserved for the discussion.

Information about the sample should address person, place, and time.

What are the general characteristics of the sample?
What is the sampling unit (group or individual)?
Where, geographically, and when was the sample selected?
How was a sampling frame, if any, constructed?
What is the source of contact information used in the frame?
What sampling technique (i.e., probability or non-probability) was used?
How many subjects or units are included in the final sample?
What is the response rate?
If a cohort, what is the retention rate?

A description about the data collection procedure(s) should make clear the type or types of methodologies used.

Is it a combination of survey and medical testing?
Is it a medical record review?
Is it a qualitative, open-ended interview?

The methods should be described briefly as they were conducted. Methods for contacting subjects should be outlined.

Was it a mail, phone, email, or face-to-face contact?
Was it a combination of these, done in a staged manner?

Methods

1. Sample

- Mention, again, the target population.
- Discuss the sampling frame–how it was constructed.
- Describe the sampling procedure–probability or non-probablity procedures, hybrid.
- Indicate the target and actual sample size.
- Indicate the response rate.
- Describe the key characteristics of the sample–person, place, time, unit of analysis.
- Present descriptive statistics about demographic characteristics of the final sample (either here or in the results section).
- If cohort, present the retention rate and descriptive statistics of demographic characteristics of those lost to the study.
- Limit to about one paragraph.

2. Data Collection Procedures

- Identify the data collection method(s) used (e.g., survey, medical tests, open-ended interview, record review.
- Describe the initial contact with potential subjects.
- Explain the recruitment procedure (e.g., mail, phone, email, in-person).
- Address the issue of IRB approval for human subjects studies.
- Limit to one paragraph.

3. Measures

- Focus primarily (or only) on the measures analyzed in the current report.
- Identify the type(s) of measures to be analyzed (e.g., survey items, biological tests, diagnoses).
- Briefly describe the key measurement procedures (e.g., assumptions, criteria, equipment, definitions, methods).
- Indicate the proportion of subjects with missing data on key measures.
- Limit to half a paragraph.

4. Analysis Procedures

- Indicate the analytic methods used in the report (e.g., meaures of association, regression, survival).
- Mention the statistical analysis package used (if appropriate).
- Limit to half a paragraph.

FIGURE 11–4 Recipe for the Methods Section

Recruitment procedures should be mentioned. Generally, what were potential subjects told about the study when they were asked to participate?

Finally, institutional review board (IRB) approval or an exemption or waiver should be indicated. Again, consider the information a reader would need to evaluate the strength of the study procedures.

The discussion about study measures or variables should focus on those that are used in the analysis reported in the present paper. It is likely that the study includes many measures not analyzed for the report, but they do not need to be described unless they are relevant, in some way, to the current analysis. The method of measurement should be mentioned if it has not already been discussed in the data collection description. Rationalize the choice and construct of the measures used. If a scale is used, cite the source of the scale (if appropriate) and briefly describe its construction. If a continuous measure is grouped into categories, discuss the assumptions used to determine the cut-points. Give some indication about the definition of the construct used to operationalize it. For example, how is self-esteem defined for the creation of the self-esteem scale? Discuss any selection criteria used, if appropriate. If some subjects are excluded from analyses based on key measures, this should be justified. Finally, missing data on key measures should be identified. If some measures cannot be used because of high proportions of missing data, this should be revealed.

At the end of this section, the analytic method(s) used for the report should be introduced. Introduce them simply by identifying them and briefly justifying their appropriateness. The justification will usually depend on the study design, variable measurements, and type of relationship (if any) examined. The statistical analysis package should also be identified and properly cited. The entire methods section should be limited to about one and a half double-spaced pages.

RESULTS

It might be surprising to the reader that the results section should be relatively short in length. It should be shorter than the introduction and the discussion sections. Obviously, it is important to present the results that support your conclusions and interpretations, but the conclusions and interpretations directly address the research question and usually cannot be communicated as succinctly as the results. In addition, the introduction should communicate the important contribution of the study, and the discussion should detail this contribution. The results should offer scientific support for the contribution.

The ingredients in the recipe of results will vary substantially from study to study. Hence, the recipe discussed here will be particularly generic. The results section has two general purposes: (1) present the numeric results, and (2) summarize and highlight them. An important part of this process is often editing. Rarely does a research report or journal article present *all* the results of the analyses conducted. The research question(s) should be answered or the hypothesis tested—supported or not supported. All results should address this purpose. Extraneous results are rarely appropriate and usually "muddy" the important contribution of the study. In fact, the results of fishing expeditions, which should not be conducted, would all be extraneous.

The numeric results should be presented in tabular or graphic form. These forms will be discussed in the next section. The tables and graphs can be embedded in the text or their position "called out" as place holders in the text. The call-outs usually look like "Table 1 About Here" and are positioned where the publisher would put the table in the article or report. The purpose of the text in this section is to put the numeric results into words. These should be straightforward statements, such as:

> "Females were 2.3 times more likely than males to be diagnosed with malignant menginomas."
>
> "There is a significant relationship ($p < 0.001$) between gender and diagnosis."
>
> "The strength of the association diminished significantly (by more than 10%) when cell phone use was included in the multivariate analysis."

Numbers and probability levels can be restated in the text, but this should be done sparingly, because this information is presented completely in the tables and graphs. Most importantly, the text should simply restate the results in words, and possibly highlight the important results. Any and all interpretation should be saved for the discussion section.

A generic recipe for the results section can include three ingredients. First are descriptive statistics of the key variables analyzed. The distribution, measure of central tendency, and/or measure of dispersion should be presented for the exposure and outcome variables, and possibly for the covariates, confounders, or effect modifiers. Second are univariate relationships (i.e., measures of association) between the exposure and outcome, and possibly other variables. Third are the multivariate models (e.g., regressions, multi-way analyses of variance [ANOVAs], survival models), including the exposure and covariates. Again, this is a generic recipe in that some ingredients may not be relevant to the purpose of the study. Generally, the results section should be limited to about two and a half double-spaced pages of text, excluding tables and graphs.

TABLES AND GRAPHS

Computer output of the analysis results is rarely, if ever, in a format that is appropriate for the report or manuscript. (Some graphic displays may be an exception.) Typically, the numeric results should be entered into tables or graphs generated in Microsoft Word or a similar word-processing package. This way, the researcher has complete control over the formatting, and specific results that are presented. The most important general comment about tables and graphs is that they should be able to stand alone—be meaningful and self-explanatory on their own if separated from the text. This requirement is accomplished by including descriptive titles, labels, scales, and footnotes.

We will start by discussing tables first. Tables should be numbered in consecutive order, such as "Table 1" and "Table 2." An example of a table of results is presented in **Figure 11–5**. This example table is meaningful without access to descriptive text about it. The title indicates where and when the study sample was selected, and the type of data for the specific variable included in the table. The column labels describe the type of data presented (frequencies and percentages), and the categories of the variable to which they apply. The note at the bottom of the table describes the construction of the variable of interest. This information is important because a measure of social support is not self-explanatory, in that it is a complex concept with multiple options for measurement. Notes should be used to present *important* information that cannot be included in the title or labels. Notes should be used sparingly and be as brief as possible. The specific data in the table should be presented consistently. The general rule for non-whole numbers is to use one or two decimal points. The choice should be used consistently.

Other common types of tables are crosstabulations, correlation matrices, and regression results. Crosstabs indicate the relationship between two or more variables. A simple two-way table shows the relationship between two variables. For an association between independent and dependent variables, the common approach to the table is to show percentage across and comparison down. The independent variable should be the row variable and the dependent variable the column. Cell percentages are calculated within the independent variable, so the "row percentage" option should be chosen in the CROSSTAB (crosstabulation) command in statistical software packages. The text summary of the table should compare percentages within categories of the dependent variable or down each column. Typically, the value and statistical significance of the appropriate measure of association are presented at

Table 1. Relative Frequency Distribution of the Social Support Scale, Chicago 1989

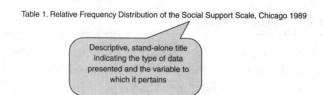

Descriptive, stand-alone title indicating the type of data presented and the variable to which it pertains

Descriptive row labels indicating the variable name and category labels

Descriptive column labels indicating the type of data, with symbols defined

Social Support	Frequency (f)	Relative Frequency (%)	Cumulative Relative Frequency (%)
Low	16	13.6	13.6
Medium	33	27.9	41.5
High	69	58.5	100.0
TOTAL	118	100.0	

Note: Social support is an aditive scale of 6 items measuring contact with and reliance on family, friends, and school colleagues. It has been recoded into 33.3% groups based on the distribution of the raw scale.

Note provides important information that cannot be communicated in the title or labels. This information allows the table to stand alone because the reader is clear about how social support is measured.

FIGURE 11–5 Table Construction

the bottom of the table, similar to a footnote. For example, the measure of association is presented like:

$$\text{chi-square} = 22.6;\ df = 3;\ p < 0.01$$

so that the reader knows the value of the measure, any relevant information such as degrees of freedom, and the level of statistical significance or nonsignificance.

Correlation matrices show the relationships between multiple continuous measures. An example matrix is presented in **Figure 11–6**. Each variable is listed as a column and as a row. A variable correlated with itself is a perfect correlation with a value of 1.00. Values listed beneath the diagonal of 1.00s are the

Table 2. Pearson Correlations Between All Independent Variables

	VAR1	VAR2	VAR3	VAR4
VAR1	1.00			
VAR2	0.82***	1.00		
VAR3	0.14	0.02	1.00	
VAR4	0.46**	0.31*	0.12	1.00

Note: * $p < 0.05$; ** $p < 0.01$; *** $p < 0.001$.

FIGURE 11–6 Example Correlation Matrix

correlation coefficients between all pairs of variables. Statistical significance of the coefficients is indicated with asterisks, the key for which is presented in the table note. This is a fairly standard method for showing statistical significance in tables that cannot accommodate p-values or confidence intervals.

An example table of logistic regression results is presented in **Figure 11–7**. This is real data presented by one of the authors at a conference. The title describes the data source and the statistics presented in the table. The table note describes how the variables are coded so that one category is the reference to which all other categories are compared. Odds ratios rather than log coefficients are presented because these are the statistics that are interpreted in the text. In epidemiologic research, confidence intervals are more commonly reported than are p-values. A confidence interval containing a value of one (1) indicates an odds ratio that is not statistically significant. Generally, one or the other group of results should be reported, not both. Present either the regression coefficients and p-values, or the odds ratios and confidence intervals. These results show that the strongest significant correlates of receptive syringe sharing (i.e., using a needle that was first used by another) with all other variables held constant are relative closeness of the injection partner, peer and personal norms about the risk of needle-sharing, and reliability of the source of clean syringes.

The construction of figures is similar to that of tables in terms of the essential use of descriptive titles and labels, and possibly footnotes. Figures should not repeat information presented in tables and vice versa. The example frequency distribution table and histogram included in this chapter should not both be presented in a report because they show the exact same data. The example

Table 3. Multivariate Correlates of Receptive Syringe Sharing: Drug Use Intervention Trial (DUIT), Baltimore, Chicago, Los Angeles, New York, Seattle, 2003 ($n=3{,}132$)

Correlate	Odds ratio	95% CI
Thrown out of house before 18	1.2	1.0–1.5
Traded sex	1.4	1.1–1.8
Place injected most (home)	1.0	
Public place	1.4	1.0–1.8
Car	1.4	1.1–1.8
Shooting gallery	1.6	1.3–2.0
Person injected with (sex partner)	1.0	
Shooting partner, friend, relative	0.6	0.5–0.8
Other	0.5	0.4–0.7
Peer norm about sharing (against)	1.0	
Neutral	2.8	2.2–3.5
Not against	2.9	2.3–3.7
HIV risk for sharing likely	0.6	0.4–0.7
Syringes mostly from needle exchange/pharmacy	0.7	0.6–0.8
Total psychiatric problems (not at all)	1.0	
A little bit	1.4	1.1–1.8
Moderately	1.8	1.4–2.4
Quite a bit/extremely	1.8	1.2–2.5
Daily injection	1.4	1.1–1.7

Note: The reference category for correlate variables with more than two categories is indicated in parentheses (and odds ratios of 1.0). The reference category for dichotomous variables is the null category. For example, the reference category for "Daily injection" is frequencies of injection less than daily.

FIGURE 11–7 Example Logistic Regression Results

Source: Data from Bailey, S. L., Ouellet, L. J., Mackesy-Amiti, M. E., Golub, E. T., Hagan, H., Hudson, S. M., Latka, M. H., Gao, W., Garfein, R. S., DUIT Study Team. (2007, November). Perceived risk, peer influences, and injection partner type predict receptive syringe sharing among young adult injection drug users in five U.S. cities. *Drug Alcohol Depend, 91*(1):S18–29. Epub 2007, April 16.

histogram is presented in **Figure 11–8**. For many figures, the sample size is presented in the title because this information is not always included in the context of the figure. A key of different colors, shades, or patterns is used to indicate the variable category each bar represents. An appropriate scale is used

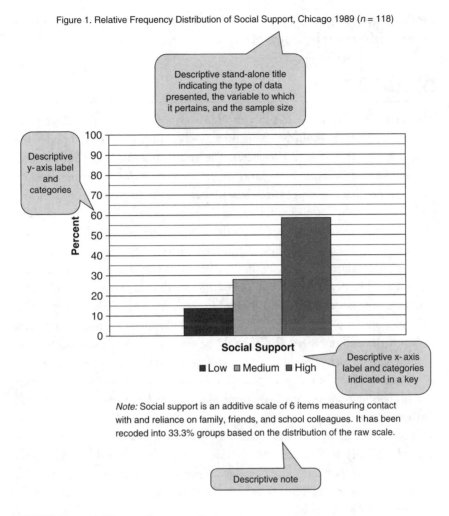

Figure 1. Relative Frequency Distribution of Social Support, Chicago 1989 (*n* = 118)

FIGURE 11–8 Figure Construction

for the y-axis. Because these are percentages with a sizeable range between them, the appropriate scale is 0 to 100, with intervals of 5 percentage points. This scale adequately represents the conceptual importance of the differences between categories. Other common figures reported in statistical studies are bar graphs, line graphs, box plots, and scatterplots. Most statistical packages can generate figures that can be imported (and possibly modified) into word-processing packages. The figures presented in this chapter were generated directly in Microsoft Word. No matter how the figure is generated, it must be clearly labeled and described so that it can stand alone meaningfully without the text of the report or manuscript.

DISCUSSION

The discussion section is arguably the most important section of the report. A complete section would be about three double-spaced pages (and preferably more if space can be spared elsewhere). The general purpose is to draw together the entire report and put the results in the context of answering the research question and directing other researchers to the possible next steps in the scientific process. Generally, the recipe for the discussion section calls for four ingredients: (1) restatement of the study hypothesis or research question, (2) summary and interpretation of the key results, (3) limitations or weaknesses of the study, and (4) implications of the study findings. **Figure 11–9** lists and describes these ingredients. The discussion section often begins with a statement like, "The purpose of this study was to." This beginning serves to remind the reader of the research question or hypothesis. Great care should be taken to choose the results to summarize and interpret. These should be directly relevant to the question or hypothesis. The focus should be on the conceptual and practical *meaning* of the results, not the specific numbers. These have already been presented in the results section. Speculations about the meaning and reasons for unexpected results are also appropriate here.

Speculations about the unexpected can lead to a discussion about the limitations of the study. It is the researcher's ethical obligation to reveal the weaknesses of the study and speculate or demonstrate, if possible, how these might affect the results. Potential or actual biases and ways that they have been minimized should be the focus in this section.

The implications of the results are the reason for doing the study in the first place.

- What do the results add to what is already known in the specific field of inquiry?
- What do the results suggest for the next steps in inquiry in this field?
- How can additional studies overcome some of this study's limitations?
- Are there caveats that should be considered in the interpretation of the results?
- How can the results be used to design evidence-based intervention or prevention programs?
- What direction should these programs take?

Discussion

1. The Research Question or Hypothesis
- Begin with a phrase like, "The purpose of this study was to…"
- Very briefly describe the important details of the study (usually the sample and data collection method).
- Restate the research question or hypothesis.
- Generally indicate whether the hypothesis was supported or the question answered.
- Limit to one paragraph.

2. Summary and Interpretation of Results
- Summarize the results that are directly relevant to the question or hypothesis.
- Avoid too much detail and repetition of the results section.
- There is no need to repeat the specific numeric results.
- Focus on the meaning not the numbers of the results.
- This is the place to speculate about what the results mean in the broader context of the area of the study.
- It is also appropriate to speculate about the reason(s) for unexpected results.
- Limit to about one page.

3. Limitations of the Study
- Here is the place to meet one aspect of our ethical duty.
- All important study weaknesses should be revealed or emphasized.
- Examples include low response rate, selection bias, insufficient statistical power, and so on.
- Efforts to address the effect of the limitations on the results should be made.
- For example, characteristics of subjects lost to follow-up should be included in models predicting the outcome.
- Informed speculations about the effect of the limitations should be made.
- Limit to about three-quarters of a page.

4. Implications of the Results
- Describe the implication of the results for the field of study.
- Suggest future studies that overcome this study's limitations.
- If relevant, describe the practical implications of the results for public health practice (treatment or prevention).

FIGURE 11–9 Recipe for the Discussion Section

The purpose of this last section of text is to link the present study to prior and future knowledge. Ideally, the results should be used in the practice of public health. This point should be clearly stated and emphasized.

CITATIONS AND REFERENCES

If the material included in the report is not common knowledge in the field or is the specific results of a particular study, then the study should be cited and referenced. Verbatim wording should be avoided and minimized, but if used, it should be enclosed in quotations and the page number where it can be found in the source should be included in the citation. Plagiarism is a violation of the researcher's ethical responsibility, and any questions about "gray areas" should be pursued and resolved. Even paraphrasing can be plagiarism. A journal's reputation is too important for there to be *any* tolerance for any type of plagiarism. Funders and educators will also not tolerate this violation of ethics.

Citations and references are an important aspect of the report where the required style should be known to the researcher/author. Several referencing packages such as EndNote and RefWorks are available for searching and formatting citations. In public health, the most commonly used style for citations and references is the American Medical Association's style guide. Current guidelines can be found in the *AMA Manual of Style, 10th Edition* (Iverson, Christiansen, Flanagin, et al., 2007). AMA style uses superscript numbers as citations in the text. The references are then numbered and listed in consecutive order as they are cited in the text. Standard abbreviations for journal titles should be used. These are indicated in the manual. Citations for online journals should include the DOI (digital object indicator) number. The citation should include the date an online article is viewed if it does not have a number or webpage. Unpublished works and personal communications should be indicated in parentheses in the text and not in the reference list.

Article and book authors are indicated by their last name and initials without periods or commas (e.g., Bailey SL). Multiple authors are separated by commas. All authors should be listed if six or fewer; otherwise the first three should be listed and followed by "et al." Journal and book titles are written in italics.

These are just a sampling of the AMA guidelines for citations and references. Most journals indicate their required style in the "Information for Authors" section, and some give examples of styles that may deviate from the norm. Specific fields also use particular styles in the requirements for theses and dissertations. The graduate school administration can be a resource for such information. Funders should also be queried about their preferred style. Other styles sometimes used in public health include the International Committee of Medical Journal Editors (ICMJE), National Library of Medicine (NLM), and American Psychological Association (APA). The required style should be known and consulted before writing begins. Fewer things are more frustrating than having to revise an incorrect style.

TITLE AND ABSTRACT

These components can only be written after the rest of the report or manuscript is complete. They are the "hooks" to catch the interest of potential readers. Like the rest of the report, they should be short and to the point. The title should be limited to about 10 to 12 words. The words should indicate the general study design and key results of the study. Information about the general study design can include key characteristics of the sample (e.g., gender, age, health status, geographic location) and type of study (RCT, cohort, cross-section). Information about study results can look like these examples: "effective trial," "X is associated with Y," or "no association between X and Y." Ineffective trials and nonsignificant relationships are worthy of publication and should be reported proudly. Journals should avoid what's called publication bias by only publishing studies with significant results, even when the study may have some serious weaknesses. In any event, the title should include important keywords that readers might use in literature search engines. Using the appropriate relevant words in the title will help assure that the publication will be identified by interested parties.

The abstract should be limited to about 120 to 180 words. It can be either structured (with headings) or unstructured (with no headings). Whether structured or unstructured, the abstract should include information about the purpose of the study, the methods used, the key results, and the conclusion based on the results. Again, important relevant keywords should be used in the abstract to help the publication to be identified in related searches. Like the report itself, more words should be allotted to the conclusion than to other parts of the abstract.

The purpose should be about one sentence, such as: "This study examined the effects of needle exchange use on syringe sharing among young injection drug users." In about two sentences, the methods should indicate the characteristics of the sample (who, where, when), the general study design, and perhaps limited information about the data collection procedures and measures. Results should be limited to the key or most important findings. Specific numbers may or may not need to be included, but level of significance ($p < 0.001$) is almost always included. Easily interpreted measures of association (e.g., odds ratios) are often included. This section should be limited to about two sentences. Finally, the conclusion should include the key interpretation and implication of the results. The meaning and use of the results can be the true "hook" to entice the reader to request the full-text article for more details. This section can be about three sentences.

ACKNOWLEDGMENTS

This information is often included in the end matter of a journal article or the front of a report or dissertation. It is important to recognize the people who "really made this possible." Aside from coauthors, who contributed significantly to the conduct of the study? If the report analyzes secondary data, then the investigators that collected the data initially should be acknowledged. Key personnel for the collection and analysis of primary data (e.g., interviewers, field managers, statisticians) should be recognized here and not included as coauthors unless they authored significant portions of the manuscript. Study funders should be noted, including the agency and grant or contract number. Finally, manuscript reviewers, both known and anonymous, should be recognized and thanked for their time and effort.

CONSORT AND STROBE

CONSORT and STROBE are two long-standing initiatives mandated to encourage the transparency and improve the quality of reporting the results of epidemiologic studies. CONSORT (Consolidated Standards of Reporting Trials) was developed in 1996 by a committee of researchers and was revised in 2001 and again in 2010 (Schulz, Altman, & Moher, 2010). CONSORT guidelines focus on the quality of reporting the results of randomized controlled trials. STROBE (Strengthening the Reports of Observational Studies in Epidemiology) is a similar committee-driven initiative focusing on the transparency and quality of reporting the results of observational studies (cohort, case-control, and cross-sectional) (von Elm, Altman, Egger, et al., 2007). STROBE was first convened in 2004.

Both initiatives released and widely published "statements" consisting primarily of checklists of information to include in research reports. Checklist items cover the main components of each section of the report—title and abstract, introduction, methods, results, discussion, and other relevant information (e.g., source of funding, trial registry). The STROBE statement includes checklists for each of the three types of observational study designs—cohort, case-control, and cross-sectional. The intent of the checklists is the honest treatment of the checklist items in published reports of research results.

Examples of items in the STROBE checklist are:

Title and Abstract	Indicate the study's design
Introduction	
Background/rationale	Explain the scientific background
Objectives	Include hypotheses
Methods	
Study design	Present key elements of the design early in the paper
Participants	Depending on the design, give eligibility criteria, etc.
Variables	Clearly define all
Data sources/measurement	Give sources of data for each variable
Bias	Describe any efforts to address sources of bias
Study size	Describe power analysis or other method to determine n
Quantitative variables	Explain how handled (e.g., recoded, scaled) in analysis
Statistical methods	Include methods to address confounding
Results	
Participants	Report number at each stage of analysis
Descriptive data	Give characteristics of study participants
Outcome data	Report numbers of outcome events
Main results	Give unadjusted estimates and, if applicable, adjusted
Other analyses	For example, analyses of subgroups and interactions
Discussion	
Key results	Summarize with reference to study objectives
Limitations	Report sources of bias/imprecision and potential effects
Interpretations	Give cautious interpretations relative to limitations, etc.
Generalizability	Discuss the external validity
Other information	
Funding	Give the source of funding and role of funders

CONCLUSION

"Short and to the point" and "just the facts" are the key phrases for this chapter. Any statement made about a relationship or effect or success of a trial *must* be supported by numeric results. Speculations should be clearly identified as just that—conclusions that are not supported by results. Following tangents at any point in the report will likely involve the use of statements that are not supported by results. Tangents add unnecessary length to the document that often has precious little space available to it. There was a scene in the film *A River Runs*

Through It where a young man wrote a short document for his father. His father read the first draft and said "go make it shorter." He gave this command after each of several drafts until the document was just a few sentences long. This is sage advice for a research report so that only the important and relevant information is presented.

The document must also reflect the ethical obligation of the investigator(s). Ethical violations include plagiarism, hidden study limitations, falsification of data, and conclusions made without support. These violations are disrespectful

Research and Practice Articles

Manuscripts should be no more than 3,500 words in the main text. Structured abstracts should be no more than 180 words, excluding headings. No more than 4 tables/figures should be included. The main text must have separate sections for the Introduction, Methods, Results, and Discussion.

Title Page

The title page should include the title of the manuscript only.

Structured Abstracts

Structured abstracts should include 4 headings: Objectives, Methods, Results, and Conclusions.

References

All references should be formatted according to the *AMA Manual of Style, 10th Edition*.

Tables and Figures

Each table and figure should be self-contained. The titles should be fully comprehensible without reference to the main text, as should any terminology or variable within the main body of footnote of the table or figure. Long tables (i.e., more than 3 manuscript pages) should be separated into 2 or more tables.

FIGURE 11–10 Excerpts from the *American Journal of Public Health* Information for Authors

Source: Benjamin, G. C., MD, FACP, FACEP (Emeritus), Executive Director of the American Public Health Association. What AJPH authors should know. *American Journal of Public Health (AJPH)* Instructions for Authors.

to the study subjects, staff, funders, educators, publishers, and the field. They are criminal if they lead to harmful interventions or avoidance of effective interventions.

The structure of the report is relatively standard—title, abstract, introduction, methods, results, tables and graphs, discussion, references, and acknowledgements. The stylistic requirements may vary according to the type of report and the targeted journal. The "Information for Authors" should be consulted before writing begins. Excerpts from the information for authors for the *American Journal of Public Health* are presented as an example in **Figure 11–10**. In many cases, the recipes for sections of the report presented in this chapter are generic. It can be thought of as a recipe for Irish stew that gives the basic ingredients (onion, carrots, celery, beef, stout, flour, beef stock, bay leaf, salt, pepper) and procedures (coat the meat with flour, brown the meat, sauté the vegetables until soft, add the liquid and bay leaf, simmer for 2 hours) but substitutions (lamb, red wine, leeks, turnip, rosemary) and changes (simmer for 3 hours) can be made. The experienced researcher, like the seasoned chef, will be able to adapt the recipes for his or her specific purpose, study design, and audience.

VOCABULARY

Abstract	Citation	Keywords
Call-outs	CONSORT	STROBE

REFERENCES

Bem, D. J. (2004). Writing an empirical research article. In J. M. Darley, M. P., Zanna, & H. L. Roediger, III (Eds.), *The compleat academic: A career guide.* (2nd ed.). Washington, DC: American Psychological Association.

Iverson, C., Christiansen, S., Flanagin, A., et al. (2007). *AMA manual of style: A guide for authors and editors* (10th ed.). New York: Oxford University Press.

Schulz, K. F., Altman, D. G., & Moher, D. (2010). CONSORT 2010 statement: Updated guidelines for reporting parallel group randomised trials. *Journal of Pharmacology & Pharmacotherapeutics, 1*(2), 100–107.

von Elm, E., Altman, D. G., Egger, M., Pocock, S. J., Gotzsche, P. C., Vandenbroucke, J. P., et al. (2007). The strengthening the reporting of observational studies in epidemiology (STROBE) statement: Guidelines for reporting observational studies. *Epidemiology (Cambridge, Mass.), 18*(6), 800–804.

CHAPTER 12

Getting Accepted: Funding, Presentation, Publication

LEARNING OBJECTIVES

- Distinguish between different forums for data dissemination.
- Draft a research proposal.
- Draft posters and oral presentations for a professional meeting.
- Explain the steps for publishing a manuscript.

CHAPTER OUTLINE

   I. Introduction
  II. Funding
 III. Presenting Results
 IV. Publishing Results
  V. Conclusion
 VI. Vocabulary
VII. Study Questions and Exercises

Don't hold on to your research findings; share them.

INTRODUCTION

This chapter discusses the main objectives in preparing proposals for funding, presentations at meetings, and manuscripts for professional journals. Funding is essential for conducting research projects, and writing proposals is the only way to obtain funding. The funding proposal should be targeted to the appropriate agency (e.g., a study of brain tumors may be funded by the National Cancer Institute) and can be in response to a specific request for a proposal (RFP) or general program announcement (PA). The process of funding is usually accomplished before the initiation of a study and sometimes after obtaining initial findings from pilot studies.

When a study is completed, research results are presented at professional meetings and published in professional journals. This process is referred to as the "dissemination of findings," or the process of sharing results with other professionals in the field of study. Data can be presented in the form of abstracts, posters, research articles, and so on. The purposes of disseminating results are to get the word out about novel information about the health phenomenon of interest, stimulate additional research, and support or refute the potential or actual efficacy of new interventions and treatment. There should be practical and/or conceptual implications from study results.

FUNDING

To conduct a research study, funding (in terms of dollars, supplies, equipment, resources, staff, etc.) is vital. Funding is obtained by submitting strong and carefully prepared proposals that outline the major aspects of the study design. Perhaps the majority of time is spent on background research concerning what is known about the health phenomena and what needs to be discovered, study designs and details that have and have not worked in the past, and practical information about the availability of resources and experience that maximize the probability that the study will be successful. All the important details should be described and justified to convince the funding review committee that the proposed study is worth funding (Monsen & Van Horn, 2008). **Figure 12–1** illustrates the general steps involved in the process of getting funded.

Proposal Preparation

The first step is background preparation and planning for the proposal. Literature reviews serve several purposes in conceptualizing the proposal: (1) demonstrating

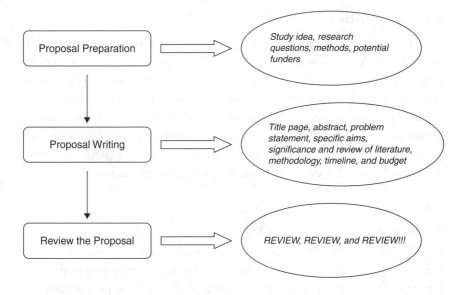

FIGURE 12–1 Steps Involved in Funding Process

the significance of the proposed study, (2) indicating the potential contribution of the new research, and (3) justifying the selection of study design, measures, and other details. A review of previous studies also helps identify study staffing needs and appropriate collaborators and reviewers. Most importantly, the review provides information necessary to refine, focus, and figure out how to operationalize the research question.

Another important aspect of prepping for the proposal is choosing a potential funder or funding agency. On most occasions, proposals are written in response to a request for applications (RFA), whereas, sometimes, seeking potential funders is also important. Knowing the requirements and focus of the funding agency is essential. Before you start writing your proposal, call the program staff (staff responsible for grants) to figure out their interest in your topic. Establish networks or use current contacts to set up networks at these funding agencies. Contacts can help garner some support for the proposal. Many times agencies offer webinars prior to proposal due dates. It is essential to attend these webinars, as they provide information regarding the types of research projects targeted for funding. Information about application materials, submission dates, specific formatting requirements, and some hints on proposal development is also covered in these webinars (Monsen & Van Horn, 2008).

Proposal Writing

Proposal writing requires perseverance, steadfastness, and strict attention to detail. The proposal should follow the funding agency's submission and preparation guidelines to the letter. One of this text's authors once had a 25-page, multi-million-dollar proposal returned without review because it had too many lines of text per inch. Beyond the specific guidelines, the proposal should clearly and accurately represent the proposed project. Components for most types of proposals include the title page, abstract, problem statement, specific aims or objectives, significance, review of literature, methodology, timeline, budget, and personnel information.

Title Page

This is a one-page document that simply provides the project title. The title should be concise, but still descriptive of the study focus, purpose, and design. It should include the keywords related to the topic being proposed. Such keywords will be made available for search if the study is funded. Specific guidelines for preparing the title page should be followed to the letter. Some guidelines require contact information for all the research investigators and some ask for information for only the principal investigator (Burns & Grove, 2005; Monsen & Van Horn, 2008).

Abstract or Summary

The abstract presents a complete overview of the proposed project in a brief and concise format. Follow the guidelines for page limit or word limit for the summary. Typically, this section of the proposal is written last, after the study design is fully developed.

Problem Statement

This section may be the most important part of the proposal in that its purpose is to justify the value of the study and provide background for the proposed research questions and hypotheses. A very brief review of the literature can be included here to justify the need for the proposed study. The problem should also align with the goals and objects of the sponsoring agency.

Specific Aims

This section provides specific aims or detailed goals of the proposed project. Depending on the study design, research questions/objectives or hypotheses should be fully explained within the aims. Here, and in the rest of the proposal, the aims should be directly and clearly relevant to the problem statement and overall purpose of the study.

Significance and Review of Literature

This section summarizes the designs and results of relevant studies and provides support for the relevance of specific aims. The breadth, relevance, and quality of the review also serve to demonstrate researchers' understanding, familiarity, and expertise in the particular field of study. Summarizing relevant studies conducted by the research team will help demonstrate this expertise. Copies of published study results should be included in an appendix. It is important to emphasize how the proposed project will extend previous research and contribute essential findings to the literature and the field in general.

Methodology

This section carries the most weight (in terms of score) in the review process. Details about the research design, subjects, data collection techniques, and data analysis should be clearly and completely explained in this section. Figures that visually explain study details are helpful and appropriate for this part of the proposal. Elements to include in the description are information on the target population, screening criteria and process, sampling, recruiting and retention, measures, data collection techniques, data processing, storage and access, power analysis justifying the proposed sample size, and analysis plan. Potential article and report titles also can be included in the analysis plan. Here, and sometimes in a special section, details about human subjects protection and institutional review board (IRB) review should be clearly and completely explained. Risks and benefits should be indicated and weighed relative to one another. Draft informed consent forms or scripts should be included in an appendix (Burns & Grove, 2005; Monsen & Van Horn, 2008).

The measures and variables should be described and justified. For example, if measuring weight, provide information on what tool will be used to collect data and in what form (pounds or kilograms). Justification for each data collection tool, including relevance and any known validity and reliability measures, should be provided.

The procedures component of the methodology section indicates the detailed and sequential steps in data collection and processing. Examples of types of information to include are: who will develop the data abstraction tool, how will it be developed, how will it be tested, who will collect the data, how will they be trained, what collection procedures will be used, where will the data be collected and over what time period, how will the data be recorded, who will enter the data into a database for analysis, and how the data will be stored and protected. The last component of the methodology is statistical analysis. In this subsection, results of the power analysis should be presented, specific statistical procedures and software should be identified and explained, and analysis personnel (e.g., the biostatistician) should be identified. The analysis plan should be presented in the context of the specific aims, and the ways in which the plan addresses the aims described in detail (Burns & Grove, 2005; Monsen & Van Horn, 2008).

Timeline

The timeline indicates to the reviewers the possibility and likelihood of completing all phases of the study in the time period requested for funding. A graphic presentation of this information is extremely helpful. The timeline should name and define each step in the research process (e.g., IRB review) and how long each will take to complete relative to the proposed start date and period of funding.

Sample Timeline

Proposed Plan	Dates
IRB approvals	August 2007
Baseline data collection (pretests, plate waste/production records, heights and weights)	September 2007
Intervention period (gardening, providing cafeteria food, nutrition/mindfulness lessons)	September 25, 2007–June 15, 2009
Post-data collection	June 15–30, 2009
Data analysis	July–August 2009

Budget and Budget Justification

The budget is an important component of the proposal. Reviewers take a look at it to evaluate the practicality of the budget relative to the goals and procedures of the study. Ideally, someone with experience preparing budgets can be consulted to help with this preparation. Universities often have grant officers to help with this part of the proposal. The budget should include dollar amounts and a detailed explanation of their use for each step of the study. The justification piece is intended to explain or justify why each step requires the specific amount of money requested. For example, the budget estimates that $2,000.00 is needed for a student worker and the justification further itemizes this expense, such as one student at the rate of $8.00/hour for 250 hours = $2,000.00.

The majority of funding agencies have their own criteria for the total amount to be funded and dates for the fiscal year. Typically, a budget form is provided by the agency in the submission packet. The form is usually divided into direct and indirect costs. Direct costs include personnel salaries and benefits, materials and supplies, equipment, travel, and consultant fees. Indirect costs are paid to the institution that hosts the primary investigator. Some institutions have negotiated a set rate (%) of total direct costs for research studies. Not all funding agencies will pay the requested indirect costs (Burns & Grove, 2005; Monsen & Van Horn, 2008).

Sample of Budget and Budget Justification

Cost	Amount
Personnel	$XXX.XX
Subject Compensation (50 participants × $25.00 = $1,250)	$1,250.00
Travel for conducting interviews	$2,500.00
Student assistance for transcription ($ 7.50/hour for 5 weeks at 10 hours per week for 1 student)	$375.00
Total	*$4,125.00*

Compensation: The interviews will last 1–2 hours. Thus, $25.00 will be given to compensate subjects for their time and willingness to participate in the study.

$$50 \text{ participants} \times \$25.00 = \$1,250$$

Travel: This study is labor intensive. Data collection will require extensive statewide travel. On average we are estimating each trip at approximately 100 miles (depending on location): 100 miles × $0.50 = $50.00 (per trip)

$$\$50.00 \times 50 \text{ participants} = \$2,500.00$$

Student Assistance: One undergraduate student will be employed for assistance with transcribing the interviews. Payment will be $7.50/hour for 1 student assistant for approximately 5 weeks and 10 hours/week.

$$\$7.50 \times 50 \text{ hours} = \$375.00$$

Personnel

Personnel are people involved in conducting the duties related to the research project. Project directors, project manager, research assistants, graduate student assistance, hourly student employees, secretary, and biostatistician are all concerned research personnel. The proposal needs to specify the exact role and time commitment of each person involved in the project. Salary is determined based on hourly cost or calculated as a percentage of salary. The majority of the budget is spent on personnel salaries (Monsen & Van Horn, 2008).

When a draft of the entire proposal is complete, it should be reviewed by persons with appropriate experience and expertise (e.g., coinvestigators, consultants, advisers, university grant personnel). Developing a strong proposal can take months, so time should be built in for review and revision. Verify that all the guidelines are followed, and gather the essential paperwork and/ or signatures of institutional representatives as needed. The key to successful grant writing is to plan ahead, set deadlines throughout the process, and revise and revise. **Figure 12–2** lists some proposal writing tips that experienced grant writers have used.

PRESENTING RESULTS

The research process does not stop after the data are collected. Disseminating research findings is an essential step in the scientific process. Findings from original research can be presented in a number of ways: abstracts, posters, oral

o Use short, simple sentences.
o Write in active voice.
o Use headings and subheadings to guide the readers.
o Use bold type in headings to attract attention.
o Use tables, graphs to break up print pages.
o Use left-margin justification. Leave the right-margin unjustified.
o Make sure there are good transitions between sections.
o Follow directions as stated in the application.
o Plan ahead and set deadlines.
o Have your peers review the proposal.
o Be ready to edit the proposal many times.

FIGURE 12–2 Proposal Writing Tips

Source: Material adapted from Monsen, E. R., & Van Horn, L. (2008). *Research: Successful approaches*. Chicago, IL: American Dietetic Association.

presentations, and manuscripts for publication in professional journals. Which method is used to present results depends on their significance, the intent of the researcher, and the interested audience. **Figure 12–3** illustrates the options.

Abstracts

Abstracts are concise summaries of the research project that serve as an introduction for journal manuscripts, oral presentations, or poster sessions. The summaries are used as brief communication tools to convey research findings to collaborators, stakeholders, and funding agencies. The organizational structure of an abstract is similar to a longer manuscript, but focuses only on important information. Abstracts are usually limited to a small number of words. Though it is very brief, the abstract should provide a clear picture of the study purpose, methods, key results, and important implications.

Writing an abstract is a skill that improves with practice. It is often challenging to present a lot of information in approximately 250 words. It takes a number of drafts to fit the needed information within the word limit. It is helpful to ask for help with editing and proofing the abstract. The researcher has to be able to highlight the most pertinent findings and present them sufficiently within the specified word count (Monsen & Van Horn, 2008).

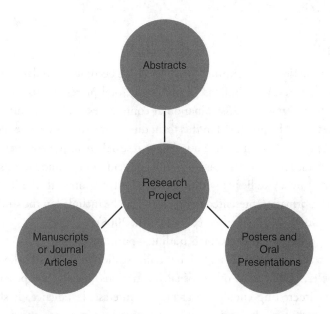

FIGURE 12–3 Most Commonly Used Methods of Disseminating Research Findings

Example of an Abstract Submitted for a Conference Presentation

Four Decades of Content Analysis of Food Advertisements on Prime-Time, Network Television

Learning Outcome: Identify the changes in food advertising on prime-time, network television across the previous 4 decades. The purpose of this study is to analyze 4 decades of television food advertisements on prime-time, network television. One hundred seven hours of television were recorded using a 3-week average of Nielsen Media Research's list of top 10 weekly shows. Content analysis was conducted for 531 food advertisements recorded from March through May 2008. Data collected were compared to food advertisement content analysis studies from previous years including: 1971, 1977, 1988, 1992, 1998. Food advertisements were classified according to type of advertisement (food product, fast food restaurant, non-fast food restaurant), types of foods advertised (13 different categories), total advertisements (rate/hour), number of food advertisements (rate/hour), and percentage of food ads per total commercials. Statistical analyses were run using SPSS 12.0 version. Linear regression was run for the number of total commercials, food advertisements, and percentage of food ads per total commercials. Chi-square analyses were computed for the type of food advertisements and the food categories advertised. Significance was determined with a p-value of < 0.01. Significant change across the 4 decades was determined for the rate of total commercials per hour ($p = 0.03$). Significant differences were also seen for the types of food advertisements: fast food restaurant ($p < 0.001$), sit-down restaurant ($p < 0.001$), food product ($p < 0.001$). Seven of the 13 food categories showed significant changes including: bread/cereal/pasta ($p < 0.001$), energy/soft drinks ($p < 0.001$), convenience/pizza/fast food ($p < 0.001$), candy/sweets ($p < 0.001$), coffee/tea/other ($p = 0.023$), sweeteners/condiments ($p < 0.001$), and other/supplements ($p < 0.001$).

Funding Disclosure: None

Source: Ederle, S., Handu, D. J., & Salmela, M. (2009, September). Four decades of content analysis of food advertisements on prime-time, network television. *Journal of the American Dietetic Association, 109*(9 Suppl.), A2.

Posters

Poster presentations at scientific conferences have become a popular and efficient way to present research findings. Traditionally, oral presentations were the primary method of research dissemination at conferences, and the results of only a few studies could be presented in this form due to limitations in time. Poster sessions make it possible for a huge number of researchers to present their findings at conferences. The poster is a visual graphic presentation of study results that can be examined by an audience with or without interaction with the investigator. The same information presented in oral form can be included in the study poster. (Burns & Grove, 2005; Monsen & Van Horn, 2008).

A poster follows the abstract outline—purpose of the research project, methods, results, and conclusions. The results section of the poster should make use of tables, graphs, and other visual illustrations. Ideally, the poster should be visually interesting enough to attract an interested audience. It should be colorful, clearly laid out, and should not be too busy with too much text. The information, from purpose to implications, should be presented from left to right on the poster. Some scientific conferences provide guidelines for the preparation of posters in terms of poster size and display format.

What follows is a brief description of the typical components of a poster.

Title of the study: The title should run across the top of the poster and should include the names of authors and their affiliations. The title should be short and informative so that it attracts the audience. The font size should be big enough to read from a distance of at least 3 feet.

Abstract: Whether or not an abstract should be included on the poster depends totally on the sponsoring agency. Consult the poster preparation guidelines of the sponsoring agency.

Introduction: The introduction or background information of the project is essential to encourage the audience to examine the rest of the poster. It provides the rationale for the study and a brief review of key studies. Research questions or hypotheses can be presented here.

Methods: This section should be detailed but succinct. The audience should understand the procedures used to select the sample, measure concepts, and analyze the data.

Results: This section is the heart of the poster. Results should be illustrated with graphs, tables, and figures. They should be visually interesting, self-explanatory, and clearly labeled. One or two summary bullet points can be included with each illustration.

Conclusion: A conclusion statement is essential to assure the audience that the poster was worth examining. Implications and possibilities for future research should be highlighted.

References: Guidelines differ in the requirement for references. Either way, references can be listed in a hard-copy text document that can be given to viewers who are interested in this level of detail.

Important additional suggestions for successful posters are:

1. The choice of fonts, font size, color, and layout are essential in attracting an audience. Colleagues can be asked to critique the poster as if they are walking through the poster session (typically a very large and crowded room).
2. Microsoft PowerPoint and laminated poster paper are the best tools and materials for creating a poster. Suggested formats for laying out material can also be downloaded from numerous sites and used as a guide.

3. During the poster session time, the author should be available, standing or sitting near the poster, to explain the findings and answer questions for the interested audience. Handouts of key results and contact information can be distributed as well.

Oral Presentation

Oral presentation is another format for presenting research findings. Important background knowledge for preparing the presentation includes the characteristics and expertise of the audience, and the time limit for the session. Oral presentations allow the researcher to present results in more detail than in a poster. It is helpful to begin with an outline for the presentation. Core elements to cover in an oral presentation are a brief review of literature to help the audience understand the purpose of the study, research questions or hypotheses, details about the methodology (subject selection, data collection methods, data analysis methods), details about the results, and conclusions. It is also helpful for the presenter to rehearse the presentation prior to the actual event, particularly to test limitations in time. Only key results should be presented, and the time limit should be respected to be fair to other speakers in the panel (Monsen & Van Horn, 2008).

Example of the Layout of Poster Presentation

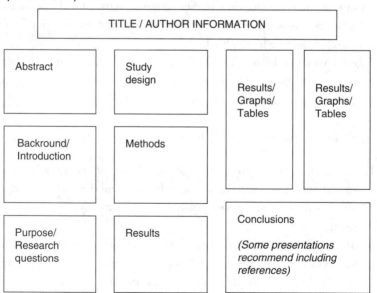

Over the years, various techniques have been used to support oral presentations. PowerPoint slides are now the preferred method of delivery. Investigators should check with the meeting sponsors to make sure a projector will be available in the meeting room. Slides can serve as an asset to the oral presentation if prepared correctly. The order of information on the slides serves as guiding tools for the flow of the presentation. Colorful graphic presentations of data should be used whenever possible. Slides should be uncluttered and free of unreadable words. Fonts should be large enough to read from the back of a reasonably sized meeting room, and lettering and background should have maximal contrast. Typically, slide backgrounds are dark (often dark blue) and lettering is light (white or light yellow). Different-colored lettering or arrows can be used to highlight important points. The slides should be carefully proofread to avoid potentially embarrassing mistakes in front of the group. Finally, the presenter may want to distribute hard copies of slides and supplemental information to interested audience members (Chatburn, 2011; Monsen & Van Horn, 2008).

PUBLISHING RESULTS

Important steps in publishing results are briefly discussed in this section.* Published journal articles can reach a large audience of researchers and practitioners. For this reason, manuscript preparation may be the most important step in the scientific method.

Choosing a Journal

Choosing the appropriate journal for the content and purpose of the article can be a daunting activity because the right choice can maximize the probability of publication. The two main issues to consider when choosing a journal are (1) the relevant journals in your field, and (2) the greatest possible access to the appropriate audience. The research topic should fit the mission of the journal. The mission is usually stated in the introductory material in each issue and the "Information for Authors." If the research is presented at a conference, then the official publication of the sponsoring agency should be consulted. It is efficient to choose the journal before writing the manuscript so that the report can be "written for the journal" in terms of format guidelines and substantive emphasis

---

*For a review of more specific details of publishing results, refer to "Reporting Results," as well as Monsen and Van Horn (2008), and Burns and Grove (2001).

(Babor, Morisano, Stenius, et al., 2008; Thompson, 2007). Important steps in choosing a journal are:

1. *Recognition factor.* Consider whether a journal is readily recognized by your peers or target audience. This increases the likelihood of being seen and read by an audience. Some of the journals have a built-in readership, as they are the official publication of the sponsoring society. Journals that are listed in Medline, PubMed, and other search engines have a higher recognition factor.

2. *Type of publication.* The focus of the research paper being submitted should be in line with the scope of the journal. Does the journal publish basic science, applied science, general public health, or specialized fields of public health? It should be the best match to the manuscript being submitted (Babor, Morisano, Stenius, et al., 2008; Thompson, 2007).

3. *Citation and impact factors.* In recent times, impact factor has become the most used standard of judging the quality of articles. Impact factors are calculated each year by the Institute for Scientific Information. They are calculated by dividing the number of times an article is cited in the previous 2 years by the total number of articles published by the journal during the same period. However, there are limitations in using this method. Different research fields have different coverage in the database; hence, journals from underrepresented fields will have low impact factors. Social sciences do not fare well on the 2-year review clock, as it is not a quickly developing research field compared to some medical areas of research, and getting cited is not an indication of the quality of research (Babor, Morisano, Stenius, et al., 2008; Callahan, Wears, & Weber, 2002; Thompson, 2007). Therefore, impact factors should be interpreted within their relevant context.

4. *Review process.* Take into consideration the time to publication and review process of the journals. The instructions to authors should be readily accessible, detailed, and should clearly state what is expected of the authors and how the manuscript will be reviewed. Journals that have a high rejection rate should specifically state the timeline for informing authors about their decision. Web-based electronic submission systems allow for an easy and efficient submission process, as well as a method for tracking the review process (Babor, Morisano, Stenius, et al., 2008; Thompson, 2007).

5. *Publishing and distribution.* It is important to know how the manuscript is presented by the journal (i.e., the layout, paper quality, how figures and

tables are printed and placed). Availability of the journal influences its visibility and accessibility. Hence, consider whether the journal is available in both print and electronic formats, and if it is listed in databases (Babor, Morisano, Stenius, et al., 2008; Thompson, 2007).

6. *Cost.* Many journals charge no fee to authors; however, there are a few that will charge either a submission fee, an acceptance fee, or cost for publishing color figures and reprints (Thompson, 2007).

Figure 12–4 presents a checklist for publishing research findings.

Components of the Manuscript

Typical components or sections for a journal manuscript are introduction, methods, results, and discussion/conclusion. The introduction should present information on prior studies, establish the problem statement, and justify the importance of the study. The methods section outlines, in reasonable detail, all the steps involved in conducting the study. It should include information on study design, subjects and their selection, data collection tools and methodology, and data analysis methods. Enough detail should be included to facilitate a replication of the study. The results section describes the major findings of the study. Results should be stated clearly and illustrated in tables or graphs. Text should not repeat all the information presented graphically. Any interpretation of the *meaning* of the results should be reserved for the discussion.

o Does the research topic fit the mission of the journal?
o Is the impact factor appropriate for the author?
o Is the journal well known in your area of research?
o Is the journal highly accessible by large number of its audience?
o Is the reviewing timeline appropriate?
o Is there an issue about cost for publishing?

FIGURE 12–4 Checklist for Publishing Research Results

Source: Material adapted from Monsen, E. R., & Van Horn, L. (2008). *Research: Successful approaches*. Chicago, IL: American Dietetic Association; Thompson, P. J. (2007). How to choose the right journal for your manuscript. *Chest, 132*, 1073–1076.

The discussion section includes a summary of key results relative to the study question or hypothesis, an interpretation of the meaning of results, the limitations of the study design and methodology, and the implications of the findings relative to past and future studies.

A review of the first draft should check that the author guidelines were followed and correct referencing format was used. Tables and graphs should "make sense" and be called out and discussed in the text. After these types of corrections, colleagues and coauthors should review the manuscript and make edits and recommendations. The manuscript should be thought of as "a work in progress" and critiques from colleagues should be accepted in the spirit of improving the quality of the paper (Monsen & Van Horn, 2008).

The last step in the process of manuscript preparation is submitting the manuscript. A cover letter is often sent with the manuscript to highlight how the manuscript is appropriate for the mission of the journal. The majority of journals have a checklist for authors that explains exactly what needs to submitted with the main manuscript. Some of the common things requested are: letter of intent, author contact information, information on copyright issues, institutional review board approval (ethics approval), tables or figures submitted separately from the main document (each table on a separate page), and the main manuscript. At present, a majority of the journals accept online submissions, which streamlines the submission process. After the submissions is final, every manuscript is assigned a tracking number, and this number is used for any further communication with the journal editors. Submission of the article initiates the process of review by editors and experts in the field (Monsen & Van Horn, 2008).

CONCLUSION

This chapter provides information and advice for obtaining research funding and disseminating results. Strong, unbiased results are only useful if they are made known to researchers and practitioners in the field. After spending huge amounts of time getting funding and conducting the study, it is worth the effort to the investigator and others in the field to prepare publishable manuscripts and powerful oral or poster presentations. These take time, energy, thought, and perspective to be well done and attractive to the target audience. The worthy benefit is to progress the field of epidemiology to the point of providing successful preventions and treatments for significant health problems in the present and future.

VOCABULARY

Abstract	Impact Factor	Timeline
Budget	Problem Statement	
Budget Justification	Proposal	

STUDY QUESTIONS AND EXERCISES

1. Draft a 250-word abstract for your study or a hypothetical study.
2. Map a poster presentation—in terms of what will be included and layout—using either your study or a hypothetical study.
3. Review an article of your choice in the *American Journal of Public Health* and briefly describe how all of the important elements of the manuscript are addressed.
4. Read and summarize the mission and information for authors in the *American Journal of Public Health.*
5. Prepare a PowerPoint slide for the title of your study or a hypothetical study. Experiment with different font types, sizes, colors, and backgrounds to determine which combinations are most readable from a distance of 3 feet.

REFERENCES

Babor, T. F., Morisano, D., Stenius, K., Winstanley, E. L., & O'Reilly, J. (2008). How to choose a journal: Scientific and practical considerations. In T. F. Babor, K. Stenius, S. Savva, & J. O'Reilly (Eds.), *Publishing addiction science: A guide for the perplexed* (2nd ed., pp. 12–36). Essex, United Kingdom: International Society of Addiction Journal Editors.

Burns, N., & Grove, S. K. (2005). *The practice of nursing research: Conduct, critique, & utilization* (5th ed.). Philadelphia: W.B. Saunders.

Callahan, M., Wears, R. L., & Weber, E. (2002). Journal prestige, publication bias, and other characteristics associated with citation of published studies in peer-review journals. *The Journal of the American Medical Association, 287,* 2847–2850.

Chatburn, R. L. (2011). *Handbook for health care research* (2nd ed.). Sudbury, MA: Jones & Bartlett.

Monsen, E. R., & Van Horn, L. (2008). *Research: Successful approaches* (3rd ed.) Chicago, IL: American Dietetic Association.

Thompson, P. J. (2007). How to choose the right journal for your manuscript. *Chest, 132,* 1073–1076.

Suggested Resources

This appendix provides additional sources of information about topics covered in text chapters.

CHAPTER 1. OVERVIEW OF THE RESEARCH PROCESS

Outline of the Research Process:

http://www.epidemiolog.net/evolving/PracticeofEpidemiology.pdf

CHAPTER 2. RESEARCH GOALS IN EPIDEMIOLOGY

Incidence and Prevalence:

http://www.epidemiolog.net/evolving/MeasuringDisease&Exposures.pdf

Measures of Association:

http://www.epidemiolog.net/evolving/RelatingRiskFactorstoHealth.pdf

Confounding:

http://www.epidemiolog.net/evolving/Multicausality-Confounding.pdf

Effect Modification:

http://www.epidemiolog.net/evolving/Multicausality-EffectModification.pdf

Validity and Reliability:

http://www.epidemiolog.net/evolving/SourcesofError.pdf

Scientific Method:

http://www.studygs.net/scimethod.htm
http://scene.asu.edu/habitat/s_method.html

Causality:

http://www.edwardtufte.com/tufte/hill
http://www.epi-perspectives.com/content/6/1/2
http://www.pitt.edu/~super4/33011-34001/33971.ppt

CHAPTER 3. OVERVIEW OF EPIDEMIOLOGIC STUDY DESIGNS

Study Designs in Epidemiology:

http://www.epidemiolog.net/evolving/AnalyticStudyDesigns.pdf
http://publichealth.jbpub.com/aschengrau/Aschengrau06.pdf
http://www.med.uottawa.ca/sim/data/Study_Designs_e.htm

CHAPTER 4. RESEARCH ETHICS

Nuremberg Code:

http://ohsr.od.nih.gov/guidelines/nuremberg.html
http://www.nejm.org/doi/full/10.1056/NEJM199711133372006

45 CFR 46:

http://ohsr.od.nih.gov/guidelines/45cfr46.html

Declaration of Helsinki:

http://ohsr.od.nih.gov/guidelines/helsinki.html

Belmont Report:

http://ohsr.od.nih.gov/guidelines/belmont.html

NIH Certification:

http://phrp.nihtraining.com/users/login.php

Guidelines for Review:

http://grants.nih.gov/grants/peer/guidelines_general/Human_Subjects_
Protection_and_Inclusion.pdf

CHAPTER 5. FORMULATING A RESEARCH QUESTION

The Research Assistant: Resources for Behavioral Science Researchers:

http://www.theresearchassistant.com/tutorial/2-1.asp

Formulating Research Questions:

http://hccedl.cc.gatech.edu/documents/115_Fisk_research%20questions%
202003.pdf
http://www.vanderbilt.edu/writing/resources/Formulating%20Your%20
Research%20Question.pdf
http://www.utexas.edu/research/pair/formulat.htm

CHAPTER 6. REVIEWING THE LITERATURE

Overview of Literature Review:

http://www.lib.ncsu.edu/tutorials/lit-review/
http://library.usm.maine.edu/tutorials/esp/sitemap.htm

Citation Software:

http://www.refworks.com/tutorial/
http://www.endnote.com/eninfo.asp

AMA Citation Style:

http://www4.samford.edu/schools/pharmacy/dic/amaquickref07.pdf

APA Citation Style:

> http://www.library.cornell.edu/resrch/citmanage/apa

Meta-Analysis:

> http://www.epidemiolog.net/evolving/DataAnalysis-and-interpretation.pdf
> http://www.cochrane.org/
> http://www.thecochranelibrary.com/view/0/index.html
> http://www.medicine.ox.ac.uk/bandolier/painres/download/whatis/
>   Meta-An.pdf

CHAPTER 7. OBTAINING SUBJECTS

Sampling:

> http://www.socialresearchmethods.net/kb/sampling.php

Recruitment and Retention:

> http://healthcare.partners.org/phsirb/recruit.htm
> http://www.appliedclinicaltrialsonline.com/appliedclinicaltrials/article/
>   articleDetail.jsp?id=89608
> http://www.wpic.pitt.edu/research/famhist/PDF_Articles/Springer/
>   RI%206.pdf

Screening:

> http://healthcare.partners.org/phsirb/prescreen.htm

CHAPTER 8. MEASURING CONCEPTS

Validity and Reliability of Measures:

> http://www.socialresearchmethods.net/kb/measure.php

Survey Measures:

> http://www.psu.edu/president/pia/innovation/Using_surveys_for_data_
>   collection_in_continuous_improvement.pdf

http://www.idready.org/courses/2005/spring/survey_IntroSurvey
Methods.pdf
http://www.cdc.gov/nchs/surveys.htm

Secondary Data:

http://sfcs.cals.arizona.edu/azsearch/sites/sfcs.cals.arizona.edu.azsearch/
files/Boslaugh,%202007.pdf

CHAPTER 9. ANALYZING DATA

Data Management:

http://www.epidemiolog.net/evolving/DataManagement.pdf
http://www.socialresearchmethods.net/kb/statprep.php

Multivariable Methods in Epidemiology:

http://www.epidemiolog.net/evolving/Multicausality-AnalysisApproaches.pdf

Data Processing:

http://www.epidemiolog.net/evolving/DataAnalysis-and-interpretation.pdf

Levels of Measurement:

http://www.epidemiolog.net/evolving/DataAnalysis-and-interpretation.pdf

Significance Testing:

http://www.epidemiolog.net/evolving/DataAnalysis-and-interpretation.pdf

Type I and II Errors:

http://www.epidemiolog.net/evolving/DataAnalysis-and-interpretation.pdf

Statistical Power:

http://www.epidemiolog.net/evolving/DataAnalysis-and-interpretation.pdf
http://power.education.uconn.edu/otherwebsites.htm
http://statpages.org/

CHAPTER 10. INTERPRETING RESULTS

General Guidelines:

Savitz, D. A. (2003). *Interpreting epidemiologic evidence: Strategies for study design and analysis*. New York: Oxford University Press.

SAS:

http://www.ats.ucla.edu/stat/sas/output/
http://support.sas.com/documentation/

Valid Interpretation:

http://www.socialresearchmethods.net/kb/concval.php

CHAPTER 11. REPORTING RESULTS

STROBE:

http://www.strobe-statement.org/

CONSORT:

http://www.consort-statement.org/consort-statement/

CHAPTER 12. GETTING ACCEPTED: FUNDING, PRESENTATION, PUBLICATION

Funding and Publication:

http://www.epidemiolog.net/evolving/PracticeofEpidemiology.pdf
http://www.aaeditor.org/StepByStepGuide.pdf

Preparing an NIH Grant Application:

http://www.theresearchassistant.com/tutorial/2-1.asp

Preparing a Poster:

http://www.eric.vcu.edu/home/resources/posters/posters_chap9.pdf

Search Engines and Public Health Sites

American Journal of Epidemiology.	http://aje.oxfordjournals.org/
American Public Health Association.	http://www.apha.org/
Annals of Epidemiology.	http://www.annalsofepidemiology.org/
CDC Wonder.	http://wonder.cdc.gov/
Centers for Disease Control and Prevention.	http://www.cdc.gov/
Epidemiology Monitor.	http://www.epimonitor.net/
Epi Info.	http://wwwn.cdc.gov/epiinfo/
	http://wwwn.cdc.gov/epiinfo/html/downloads.htm
Food and Nutrition Information Center.	http://fnic.nal.usda.gov/
Framingham Heart Study.	http://www.framinghamheartstudy.org/
Healthy People 2020.	http://www.healthypeople.gov/2020/
International Journal of Epidemiology.	http://ije.oxfordjournals.org/
Journal of the American Medical Association.	http://jama.ama-assn.org/
Lancet.	http://www.thelancet.com/

Maternal and Child Health (U.S. Department of Health and Human Services). — http://www.mchb.hrsa.gov/

Medline. — http://www.nlm.nih.gov/bsd/pmresources.html

MedlinePlus. — http://www.nlm.nih.gov/medlineplus/healthstatistics.html

Morbidity and Mortality Weekly Report (MMWR). — http://www.cdc.gov/mmwr/

National Cancer Institute. — http://www.cancer.gov/aboutnci/cis/page1

National Center for Health Statistics. — http://www.cdc.gov/nchs/

National Death Index. — http://www.cdc.gov/nchs/ndi.htm

National Health and Nutrition Examination Survey. — http://www.cdc.gov/nchs/nhanes.htm

National Health Information Center. — http://www.health.gov/nhic/

National Health Interview Survey. — http://www.cdc.gov/nchs/nhis/about_nhis.htm

National Immunization Survey. — http://www.cdc.gov/nchs/nis.htm

National Institutes of Health. — http://www.nih.gov/icd/

National Longitudinal Study of Adolescent Health. — http://www.cpc.unc.edu/projects/addhealth

National Maternal and Infant Health Survey. — http://www.cdc.gov/nchs/nvss/nmihs.htm

National Nursing Home Survey. — http://www.cdc.gov/nchs/nnhs.htm

National Survey of Family Growth. — http://www.cdc.gov/nchs/nsfg.htm

National Survey on Drug Use & Health. — http://www.oas.samhsa.gov/nsduh.htm

New England Journal of Medicine. — http://www.nejm.org/

Popline. — http://www.popline.org/

Public Health Foundation. — http://www.phf.org/Pages/default.aspx

Public Health Institute. — http://www.phi.org/

Public Health Reports. — http://www.publichealthreports.org/

Rand Health Surveys and Tools. — http://www.rand.org/health/surveys_tools.html

Substance Abuse and Mental   http://www.samhsa.gov/
  Health Services Administration.
USAID Demographic and Health   http://www.measuredhs.com/
  Surveys.
U.S. Census Bureau.   http://www.census.gov/
U.S. Department of Health and   http://www.hhs.gov/
  Human Services.
U.S. Vital Statistics System.   http://www.cdc.gov/nchs/data/
                                      misc/usvss.pdf

World Health Organization.   http://www.who.int/en/
Youth Risk Behavior   http://www.cdc.gov/healthyyouth/
  Surveillance System.   yrbs/index.htm

Exercise: Data Analysis

Included with the supporting material for this text is a data file in Excel format. For this exercise, you will need to access the data set, analyze it in Excel, or convert it to your statistical package of choice. Before you begin, you are expected to have a working familiarity with Excel or the other format you will be analyzing within. At the least, progress through the tutorials for the package you will be using. The online help menus will also be very helpful as you get started.

The data were collected via an Internet survey and include measures of health-related behaviors and demographic characteristics. Included with the data set is documentation of the data in the form of the survey instrument with associated frequencies. This is a "real" data set with warts (e.g., missing data and some weak measures) and all. Part of this exercise is learning how to make the best of what you have and decide what is impossible to do because of what you do not have.

What follows are some suggested exercises for working with these data. You are encouraged to "play around with the data" to gain experience formatting variables and running analyses.

1. Get to know the data:
   a. Run frequency distributions for each variable and compare the frequencies with those reported in the documentation to be sure you know what the numbered variable responses in the data set mean conceptually (e.g., 1 = strongly agree, etc.).
   b. Note the amount of missing data for each variable.
   c. Note the variables with less than ideal distributions (i.e., variable categories with very small frequencies).

2. Make the data yours (once you have chosen a research question):

   a. Label the variables and the response options you will be using in your analysis.

   b. Make necessary recodes based on statistical (e.g., low-frequency categories) and conceptual response (e.g., you want the scale to start with strongly disagree rather than strongly agree).

   c. Rename and label the categories of any recoded variables. Be sure to *save* them in your data file.

   d. Run frequencies for each of your recoded variables and compare them to the originals to be sure the recodes worked as you intended. Make sure all new categories are there and that their frequencies are correct. Go back and fix or redo the ones that do not look correct.

3. Choose your research question(s):

   a. What are the demographic characteristics of this sample?

   b. Do the subjects have a generally healthy diet?

   c. What are the common stages of change (transtheoretical model) for subjects in terms of their diets?

   d. What demographic characteristics are associated with a healthy diet?

   e. What is the average body mass index (BMI) in this sample?

   f. Is body image associated with BMI in this sample?

   g. Do the subjects have a generally healthy exercise routine?

   h. What demographic characteristics are associated with a healthy exercise routine?

   i. How prevalent is the consumption of fast food in this sample?

   j. What demographic characteristics are associated with fast food consumption?

   k. How prevalent is proper hand-washing in this sample?

   l. What demographic characteristics are associated with proper hand-washing?

   m. How prevalent is the practice of proactive health behaviors in this sample?

   n. What demographic characteristics are associated with proactive health behaviors?

   o. Is general health associated with proactive health behaviors in this sample?

   p. Is stress associated with proactive health behaviors in this sample?

   q. Is self-esteem associated with proactive health behaviors in this sample?

r. Are psychiatric issues associated with proactive health behaviors in this sample?

s. What other questions interest you, given the measures available in the data set?

4. Create scales for appropriate constructs, such as stress, self-esteem, psychiatric issues, general diet, exercise routine, level of health of behaviors, effectiveness of hand-washing practices, BMI, and so on.

a. Examine each item to include in the scale and recode as necessary.

b. Create the scale as appropriate (i.e., add variables).

c. Check the frequency distribution of the new scale.

d. Recode as appropriate and check again.

e. Run descriptive statistics as appropriate.

5. Run appropriate analytic techniques to address your research question(s). These may include:

a. Crosstabs with appropriate measures of association

b. Correlation matrices

c. Tests for confounding

d. Tests for effect modification

e. Multivariable analyses

6. Interpret the results of your analysis to address your research question(s).

a. Prepare tabular and/or graphic representations of your results (descriptive and inferential).

b. Summarize and interpret the results in writing.

Answers to Selected Study Questions

CHAPTER 2

1a. Descriptive goal
2a. Analytic goal, laboratory study
3a. Analytic goal, experiment study, animal study
4a. Analytic goal, clinical trial

CHAPTER 3

1a. Case-control study
3a. Cross-sectional study
5a. Cohort study

CHAPTER 5

4. A good research question should be ethical, clear, feasible, and significant. It should be feasible, interesting, novel, ethical, and relevant (FINER).
5. Descriptive
6. Descriptive

CHAPTER 6

1. Books, journal articles, and databases
2. Identify key terms using correct search strategies, select relevant and good quality research, and take notes on the key aspects of each article.
4a. Unintentional injury, intentional injury, injury-related mortality
4b. Socioeconomic status, obesity, CVD risk factors, ethnicity

CHAPTER 7

1a. Records of cigarette sales; households for survey
1b. Medical records
1c. Pharmacy records of patients taking medication for sleeping problems
1d. Patrons of needle-exchange programs
2a. Random sample of households
2b. Stratified random sample to represent important patient characteristics
2c. Random sample of pharmacists' lists
2d. Non-probability sampling such as snowball or respondent-driven sampling
4a. Schedule of delivery of practical incentives like toiletries, clothing, blankets
4b. Schedule of free medical examinations
4c. Use of school records (parents' contact information) and guidance counselor information about college and job plans; schedule of monetary incentives post–high school
4d. Daily home visits
5a. High
5b. Low
5c. Medium
5d. Medium to high

CHAPTER 8

2. *Validity* refers to the ability of the instrument to measure what it is intended to measure. Some of the common measures of validity are predictive validity, concurrent validity, convergent validity, and discriminant validity. For example, a survey tool designed to measure nutrition knowledge is used in a study to determine nutrition knowledge of college students and determine whether there is a relationship between nutrition

knowledge and food behaviors. If students with higher scores on the nutrition knowledge tool also demonstrate an increased consumption of healthy foods, then the scale is said to have high predictive value.

Reliability is the ability of the tool to yield consistent findings. Inter-rater reliability, test-retest reliability, parallel-forms reliability, and internal consistency are some common measures of reliability. For the example stated above, when the survey tool to measure nutrition knowledge was designed, the surveyor wanted to assure that the students respond to the test in the same way on repeated occasions. To test reliability of this survey, a small subset of students were assigned this survey at point 1, and then after 1 week were assigned this survey again (point 2). Statistically comparing the scores between these two points is called test-retest reliability.

CHAPTER 9

1a. Frequency distribution; bar graph
1b. Frequency distribution; histogram
1c. Mean, standard deviation; median interquartile range if skewed; linear graph
2a. Ratio, difference
2b. Chi-square test of independence
2c. Linear regression

Glossary

Abstract—summary of a study presented in a short and concise format.

Adjusted analysis—analysis of the association between an exposure and an outcome that takes into account the effects of a third variable.

Alpha (α)—the level of significance in a hypothesis test. The probability of a Type I error, or the probability of rejecting a true null hypothesis.

Alternative hypothesis (research hypothesis)—statement postulating a difference, change, association, or effect in comparisons between variables or with theoretical values. The alternative hypothesis is tested against the null hypothesis of no difference, no change, no association, or no effect.

Ambispective—looking forward and backward in time. In the context of study design, an ambispective cohort study first measures the exposure and then uses historical data to go back in time and measure prior exposure and forward in time to measure the outcome.

Analogy—criteria for causality stipulating that a causal relationship is more plausible if an association between a similar exposure and/or a similar disease has already been established.

Analysis of variance (ANOVA)—analytic procedure to test the equality of more than two independent group means.

Analytic goal—study purpose to test hypotheses concerning the factors that may be associated with or causes of an outcome.

Anonymous—data from subjects whose names are never recorded.

Assent—agreement to participate in research made by a minor or cognitively impaired individual. Consent must also be given by adults of the age of consent (e.g., parents) and/or those mandated with the best interests of the impaired individual (e.g., caretakers).

Association research goal—study purpose to determine the factors that are related to health phenomena.

Attributable risk—proportion of the prevalence or incidence of the outcome for the exposed group that can be attributed to the exposure.

Attrition bias—distortion in the association between the exposure and outcome due to a problem in the retention of subjects in a cohort or experimental study. The association between the exposure and outcome may be different for members of the baseline sample who were retained in the study from baseline to follow-up compared to baseline subjects who were lost to the study before follow-up (known as attrition).

Autonomy—subjects should enter research voluntarily and with adequate information.

Bar graph—graphic display of the frequencies or percentages of responses in categorical variables. In contrast to histograms, the bars in bar charts are separated from one another by spaces in the graph.

Belmont Report—named after the Belmont Conference Center in Elkridge, Maryland, where the committee meeting took place, was drafted and approved by the 11-member National Commission for the Protection of Human Subjects of Biomedical and Behavioral Research. The purpose of the report was to broaden and clarify the rules set forth in the Nuremberg Code, Helsinki Declaration, and the 1974 federal regulations. The report has four parts—Part A: Ethical Principles and Guidelines for Research Involving Human Subjects, Part B: Boundaries Between Practice and Research, Part C: Basic Ethical Principles, and Part D: Applications.

Beneficence—philosophy of doing mainly or only good for individuals, which is practiced in medicine and health research.

Beta (β)—the probability of making a Type II error in a hypothesis test, or the probability of failing to reject a false null hypothesis. Statistical power is $(1 - \beta)$.

Blinding—the process of keeping the study participant or investigator from knowing the treatment status (experimental or control group) of the participant.

Box-Whisker plot—a graph showing the range, first quartile, median, and third quartile for a continuous variable.

Budget—itemized summary of intended expenditures for the conduct of a study over a fixed time period.

Budget justification—description or explanation of each line item included in the budget to conduct a study.

Call-outs—place-savers in the text of a manuscript where tables and figures will be inserted during the publication process.

Case-control study—study design in which participants are selected on the basis of their outcome status. Cases are individuals with the outcome of interest, and controls are individuals who are similar in relevant ways to cases but are free of the outcome. The hypothesized exposure or risk factor is evaluated retrospectively.

Case report or study—a detailed report of the characteristics, symptoms, and other relevant information of a single patient or case.

Case series—an analytic review of the characteristics, symptoms, and other relevant information of a small group of patients or cases with similar health issues.

Categorical level—a variable measured with a fixed number of unordered response options.

Causal research goal—intention of a study to demonstrate that an outcome is the result of an exposure.

Central tendency—the average or common response or value in a variable distribution.

Chi-square (χ^2) test—a test using the χ^2 statistic that is appropriate for comparisons involving categorical variables. The calculations of the statistic involve comparing the observed data values to values that would be expected if there is no difference or no relationship between variables.

Citation—indication of the outside source (usually author and date) of a concept, result, opinion, or idea mentioned in the text of a report or manuscript.

Clinical source—places like hospitals and medical practices where cases may be located for case-control studies. A strong study design would recruit controls from the same or similar settings.

Classification Bias—see misclassification bias.

Cochran Collaboration—independent, not-for-profit organization that works to provide compiled scientific evidence to healthcare providers. They prepare, conduct, and ensure accessibility of systematic reviews in the field of health care.

Cochran-Mantel-Haenszel method—a procedure used to calculate a measure of association between an exposure and an outcome that accounts for the confounding effects of a third variable. The method is appropriate for assessing the relationship between dichotomous exposures and dichotomous outcomes. The resulting measure of association is a weighted average of the measures of association across groups or strata of the confounding variable.

Coefficient of variance—a unitless measure of variation. In ANOVA, it is the standard deviation of the error term divided by the mean of the dependent variable, multiplied by 100.

Coercion—unethical practice of forcing research subjects to participate in research studies.

Coherence—criteria for causality requiring that the association makes sense given what is known about the biology and natural history of the particular disease.

Cohort—a group of study participants defined by some common characteristic such as the same birth year, the same occupation group, and so on, who are studied over a period of time. The goal of the cohort study is to monitor the cohort over time to measure the exposures and outcomes of interest.

Community trial—experiment or evaluation design in which groups or communities are randomly (when possible) assigned to comparison groups (i.e., experimental and control) then followed to determine the presumed efficacy of the intervention.

Conceptual model—framework for the organization of knowledge of a topic of interest that helps establish a focus and serves as a guide for examining relationships between concepts (e.g., exposure, outcome, covariates, intervening factors, confounders, effect modification).

Conceptualization—process of developing an idea, especially a research idea.

Concurrent validity—ability of a measure to distinguish between groups that it theoretically should be able to distinguish between.

Confidence interval—a range of plausible values for a population parameter with a particular level of confidence (e.g., 95%) that the interval contains the true unknown parameter.

Confidential—data that is not linked to subjects' names or other identifying information. The information is collected but care is taken to keep the identifiers separate from the data.

Confounding—a distortion in the value of a measure of association between an exposure and an outcome due to the effect of a third factor or confounding variable. The confounder affects both the exposure and the outcome.

CONSORT—acronym for Consolidated Standards of Reporting Trials, which are guidelines that focus on the quality of reporting the results of randomized controlled trials.

Construct validity—degree to which individual observable measures represent the theoretical concepts they are intended to measure.

Continuous level—a variable measured with an unlimited number of responses between a defined minimum and maximum value. The response options are defined by inherently meaningful numeric values. Continuous variables are also called quantitative or measurement variables.

Control group—research subjects who are not receiving the experimental treatment or do not have the outcome of interest, but are compared to the group receiving the treatment or who have the outcome.

Convenience sample—a non-probability-based sample where subjects are selected on the basis of being conveniently available to the researcher.

Convergent validity—degree to which a measure is similar to other measures to which it theoretically should be similar.

Correlation—a measure of association that shows the magnitude and direction of the relationship between two continuous variables.

Criteria for causality—factors that are necessary or sufficient to demonstrate that an exposure causes an outcome.

Cross-contamination—threat to study validity due to subjects in the experimental group not receiving the intervention and/or subjects in the control group receiving the intervention.

Cross-sectional study design—study design in which the exposure and outcome are measured at the same point in time.

Crosstab—tabular representation of the association between two or more variables with cell sizes showing the number of subjects in each of the possible paired categories of both variables. Also a command in analytic computer software.

Crude analysis—analysis of the association between an exposure and an outcome that does not account for the effects of a third variable.

Cumulative incidence—the ratio of the number of new cases of disease during the study period to the total number of individuals who are at risk for the disease—they are free of the disease at the beginning of the study.

Database—organized collection of data for one or many purposes. There are a number of state and federal public health databases publicly available for researchers to analyze. Also, term used to describe collections of searchable sources of information.

Deception—misleading a research subject about the purpose or specific procedures of a research study.

Decisionally impaired—potential research subject who does not have the maturity, freedom, or cognitive capability to make an informed and voluntary decision to participate in a research study.

Declaration of Helsinki—the 1964 World Medical Association Declaration of Helsinki set forth ethical principles, many of which addressed the requirement of informed consent. The declaration was the first to suggest an independent committee to evaluate and monitor the ethical conduct of human subject research.

Degrees of freedom (*df*)—number of values in the final calculation of a statistic that are free to vary. For example, with one sample and one calculation (mean), there are (n – 1) degrees of freedom left to vary after the calculation of the statistic. After estimating two means in two independent samples, there are $[(n_1 - n_2) - 2]$ degrees of freedom. The specific formula for degrees of freedom depends on the particular analytic procedure.

Dependent variable—the primary response or outcome variable in an analysis. It is affected or influenced by the exposure or dependent variable.

Descriptive epidemiology—a branch of epidemiology intended to describe the relevant characteristics of a disease or other type of outcome. The disease is described in terms of person, place, and time—who has it, where it is located, and when it occurs.

Descriptive goal—research focus on describing the disease. No hypotheses are tested.

Descriptive questions—research questions focused on learning more about the characteristics of a disease. Questions are asked rather than hypotheses tested.

Determinant—factor or event that causes a change in the outcome of interest.

Deterrent—factor or event that prevents a change in the outcome of interest.

Dichotomous level—a variable measured with exactly two possible responses.

Discriminant validity—degree to which a measure is not similar to other measures from which it should be divergent.

Dispersion—variability of data points around a measure of central tendency in a frequency distribution.

Dose-response—linear relationship between the dose or exposure and response or outcome. For example, as the exposure increases, the outcome also increases.

Double blinding—the process of keeping both the study participant and the investigator from knowing the treatment status (experimental or control group) of the participant.

Dummy variable—a set of dichotomous variables used to distinguish between two or more categories. The variables are assigned values of 0 and 1, where the 0 category is the group to which the other categories are compared.

Ecologic fallacy—incorrect conclusion about the relationship between exposure and outcome on the individual level drawn for the results of a study showing an association on the group level.

Ecologic study—study design that measures the association between exposure rates and outcome rates for groups or populations. The unit of analysis in the study is the group rather than the individual.

Effect modification—situation in which the magnitude and/or direction of the relationship between the exposure and outcome differs between categories of a third variable. Also called statistical interaction.

Efficacy—capacity of a drug, treatment, device, or intervention to produce a beneficial change. Those who are exposed to the intervention do better than those who are not.

Epidemiology—study of the distribution, determinants, and deterrents of health phenomena in populations.

Estimate—likely value of a population parameter based on a sample statistic.

Evaluation—study design to test the efficacy of an intervention relative to a control condition.

Evidence-based—programs or initiatives whose designs are based on the results of relevant research.

Exclusionary criteria—subject characteristics that exclude them from study recruitment of randomization.

Experimental study—study design in which the investigator manipulates the exposure and randomly assigns subjects into a group that receives the exposure and a group that does not. Any change in the outcome is then measured.

Exposure—factor thought or shown to be predictive of an outcome or health phenomenon.

External validity—extent to which the sample is a true representation of the target population from which it is drawn.

***F* statistic**—test statistic used in ANOVA. It is the mean square model divided by the mean square error.

FINER—acronym used to define the characteristics of a good research question. F stands for feasible, I for interesting, N for novel, E for ethical, and R for relevant.

Frequency—the number of research subjects in particular groups defined by categories or values of a variable.

Generalizability—the extent to which sample results are representative of population results.

Gold standard—sufficiently tested and accepted valid measure to which new measures are compared. Also, term used to describe experimental studies that are designed with the best possible potential for minimizing research bias.

Group-level analysis—study using groups (e.g., patients at the same hospital, students at the same school) as the unit of analysis.

Guttman scale—multidimensional measure for which two or more variables are added together.

Hazard ratio—the ratio of the expected number of events per unit of time for two independent comparison groups.

Health belief model—one of the most commonly used theories to study health-related behaviors. It is based on the concept that health behaviors are influenced by personal beliefs and/or perceptions of disease and the management of disease. Theoretical concepts include perceived barriers, susceptibility, benefits, cues to action, motivating factors, and self-efficacy.

Heterogeneity—in the context of meta-analysis, refers to extent to which studies with different study designs (and types of measures of effect) are analyzed together as a group. In other words, heterogeneity is the presence of variation in true effect sizes underlying the different studies.

Histogram—a graphic display for an ordinal variable where response options are shown on the horizontal axis and frequencies or percentages are shown on the vertical axis. Bars in the graph indicate the frequency or percentage of subjects in each response group. Bars touch each other within the graph to represent the continuum in ordered response options.

HUIT—acronym of components of epidemiologic study designs that are useful for classifying and identifying designs. H is for hypothesis tested or not, U is for unit of analysis, I is for intervention tested or not, and T is for timing of the measurement of the exposure and outcome.

Hybrid designs—combination of parts or the whole of two different study designs in a new study.

Hypothesis—supposition tested by analyzing data for the purpose of supporting or not supporting its truth.

Hypothesis testing—procedure that assesses the probability that a statement made about a population parameter is true based on the calculation of sample statistics.

Impact factor—value that indicates the relative importance of an academic journal within its field. It is calculated as the average number of citations made for each paper published in that journal during the last 2 years. Journals with higher impact factors are considered to be more important compared to those with lower impact factors.

Imputation—act of assigning real values to missing data in variables. Assignments are made based on the best available information, logic, and reasonable assumptions.

Incentives—monetary or other types of gifts given to subjects for participating in a research study.

Incidence—the number of new cases of disease or some outcome during a period of time.

Incidence density (incidence rate)—the ratio of the number of new cases of disease to the total follow-up time at risk (i.e., the sum of the products of number of persons and time at risk before disease, death, or study dropout).

Inclusionary criteria—subject characteristics that are desired or needed to include them in a study.

Independent variable—the predictor, risk factor, or exposure hypothesized to predict or be associated with the outcome or dependent variable.

Individual-level analysis—study using individuals as the unit of analysis.

Information bias—systematic error in the measurement of the exposure or outcome.

Informed consent—complete disclosure of all aspects of the research; verified subject comprehension of research procedures; voluntary consent without coercion or undue influence.

Institutional review board (IRB)—groups convened at every institution where research is conducted to review study protocols and approve them only if they meet ethical standards of informed voluntary consent and benefits greater than risks.

Instrumentation—art and science of measurement.

Intention to treat—analysis strategy in which subjects are analyzed in the treatment group to which they were initially assigned regardless of whether or not they followed the study protocol completely.

Intercept (*y*-intercept)—in linear regression analysis, the value of the dependent variable (*y*) when the independent variable (*x*) is equal to zero (0).

Internal consistency—the extent to which different measures of the same construct yield similar results.

Internal validity—extent to which the sample is a true representation of the study population or sampling frame from which it is drawn.

Interquartile range—measure of variability showing range of variable values within which the middle 50% of subjects are located.

Inter-rater reliability—extent to which the measurements made by two different interviewers or researchers on the same subject are consistent.

Interval level—a type of continuous variable measured on a constant scale where the distance between adjacent values are equal across the entire scale. However, the scale does not have an absolute zero (e.g., temperature) to facilitate comparisons for values in a ratio format.

Intervention—preventative or therapeutic effort intended to have a desirable effect on health phenomena.

Justice—philosophy that classes of subjects should not, without scientific justification, be included or excluded from research; benefits from treatment should be made available to all who need it, including those who participated in the study.

Kaplan-Meier approach—popular method for calculating the survival time of subjects from study start to the event of interest, study dropout, or end of the study, whichever comes first. The method is used in cohort studies and clinical trials.

Keywords—descriptive terms that define the content of research articles and reports. The terms are used to search databases for studies on specific topics, with specific methodologies, and so on.

Kruskal-Wallis test—a nonparametric test used to compare the medians of more than two independent groups.

Kurtosis—measure of the heaviness of the tails of a distribution. Kurtosis is positive if the tails are heavier (a higher frequency) than for a normal distribution and negative if the tails are lighter (a lower frequency) than for a normal distribution.

Level of measurement—ways in which variables are measured that can be categorized into four levels of detail and amount of information ranging from lower to higher in the order of categorical (nominal and dichotomous), ordinal, and continuous (interval and ratio). The level of measurement influences the type of statistical analysis that can be performed on the variable.

Level of significance (α)—the acceptable probability of making a Type I error or rejecting a null hypothesis that is really true. The level is predetermined so that the true probability value in the hypothesis test should be less than or equal to α in order to reject the null hypothesis.

Likert scale—response options in a measure that are ordered from most to least (e.g., strongly agree to strongly disagree). Typically, there is an odd number of responses with the middle category representing a neutral position (e.g., neither agree nor disagree).

Linear regression analysis—technique used to estimate the equation that best describes the association between one or more independent or exposure variables and one continuous dependent or outcome variable.

Line graph—graphic representation of the frequencies or percentages of the distribution of categorical variables.

Logistic regression analysis—technique used to estimate the equation that best describes the association between one or more independent or exposure variables and one dichotomous dependent or outcome variable.

Mann-Whitney U test (Wilcoxon rank sum test)—nonparametric test used to compare outcomes between two independent groups to test if two samples are likely from the same population, or to determine if two populations have the same distribution shape.

Matching—selecting members of comparison groups on the basis of having similar relevant characteristics.

Matrix—table with matching rows and columns. For example, a correlation matrix shows the correlation coefficients for every possible pair of variables. Every variable has an entry as a column and as a row.

Maximum value—the largest value in a range of values.

Mean—measure of central tendency or location, computed as the ratio of the sum of a set of values of a variable to the size of the set.

Mean squares error—statistic calculated in ANOVA. It is the sum of the squared deviations of data values from their respective group means divided by its degrees of freedom. This is the denominator in the F statistic.

Mean squares model—statistic calculated in ANOVA. It is the sum of the squared deviations of group means from the overall mean divided by its degrees of freedom. This is the numerator in the F statistic.

Mean squares total—statistic calculated in ANOVA. It is the sum of the mean squares model and the mean squares error.

Median—measure of central tendency or location, defined as the value of the variable that separates the top 50% of the distribution from the bottom 50%.

Meta-analysis—systematic approach to reviewing literature that combines and analyzes data (e.g., effect sizes) from carefully chosen relevant studies conducted by other researchers. Conclusions are made from the results of the meta-analysis.

Minimal risk—"Minimal risk means that the probability and magnitude of harm or discomfort anticipated in the research are not greater in and of themselves than those ordinarily encountered in daily life or during the performance of routine physical or psychological examinations or tests" (Department of Health and Human Services. [2009]. *Code of Federal Regulations Title 45 Public Welfare, Part 46 Protection of Human Subjects*, effective July 14, 2009.).

Minimum value—the lowest value in a range of values.

Minor—individual who has not reached the legal age of consent (age 18 in the United States).

Misclassification bias—a type of information bias where subjects are incorrectly classified in groups due to problems with the definition of group criteria (e.g., definition of a case in case-control studies).

Missing data—measures for which subjects were not counted or included.

Modal instance sample—procedure to identify for the purpose of recruiting the most common "type" of subject.

Mode—a measure of central tendency or location, defined as the most frequently occurring value of a variable.

Moments—statistic summaries of a distribution in univariate analysis.

Multilevel study—research analyzing both individual- and group-level data.

Multiple regression—technique used to estimate the equation that best describes the association between two or more independent or exposure variables and one dependent or outcome variable. Multiple regression means more than one independent or exposure variable is included in the regression equation. Multiple regression can be either linear (continuous outcome) or logistic (dichotomous outcome).

Multi-stage sampling—the combined use of two or more sampling strategies.

Multivariable analysis—analysis to estimate the combined effect of two or more independent or exposure variables on a single dependent or outcome variable.

Mulitivariate analysis—analysis to estimate the combined effect of two or more independent or exposure variables on two or more dependent or outcome variables, considered simultaneously.

National Research Act—1974 act requiring researchers to obtain voluntary informed consent from subjects and establishing institutional review boards (IRBs) at universities and research facilities.

Nested case-control study—a case-control study that is developed in the conduct of another study design, usually a cohort study. Cases and controls are identified in a cohort study and recruited to participate in a case-control study.

Nominal level—a variable measured with a fixed number of unordered response options, also known as categorical level.

Nonparametric test—analytic test that is based on very few assumptions about the distribution of the variables included in the analysis, particularly the outcome variable.

Nonprobability sampling—a sampling method with which subjects are selected without using a probability-based method. The probability of selection for each subject is unknown.

Nonresponse bias—distortion in the association between the exposure and outcome due to a problem in the recruitment of subjects selected for the study. The association between the exposure and outcome may be different for members of the population who agreed to participate in the study compared to those who refused to participate.

Normal distribution—probability distribution for a continuous variable where the mean, median, and mode are equal to one another. The distribution takes the shape of a bell with symmetry around the mean. The probability distribution of z-score values is normal in shape.

Null hypothesis—statement of no difference, no change, no association, or no effect in comparisons between variables or with theoretical values. The null hypothesis is tested against the alternative or research hypothesis postulating a difference, change, association, or effect.

Nuremberg Code—directives protecting human research subjects. The guidelines were developed in 1947, following the Nazi trial of war crimes held in Nuremberg, Germany.

NY Jewish Chronic Disease Hospital Study—research conducted in 1963 where 19 critically ill (from non-cancer diseases) patients were injected with cancer cells to demonstrate natural immunity to cancer.

Odds—ratio of the number of events to nonevents, or ratio of the probability of an event to its complement (i.e., the probability of exposure to that of nonexposure).

Odds ratio—the ratio of two odds. For example, the ratio of the odds of exposure for the cases relative to the odds of exposure for the controls.

Operationalization—method of translating research concepts into observable measurements.

Oral presentation—spoken dissemination of study results directly to an audience.

Ordinal level—a variable measured with a fixed number of ordered response options. There is no measurable distance between response categories.

Outcome—the primary response or dependent variable in an analysis. In the context of epidemiology, the outcome is the health phenomenon of interest.

Outliers—values outside the range of those expected or outside the range of typical values.

Parameter—summary measure computed in a population.

Parametric test—analytic test that is based on the assumption that the outcome has a particular probability distribution and involves the estimation of parameters in that distribution.

Parental consent—consent given by a parent or guardian on behalf of a minor to participate in a research study.

Pearson correlation coefficient—measure of linear association between two continuous variables. Values range from –1.0 (perfect negative correlation) to 1.0 (perfect positive correlation).

Percentile—value in a distribution that holds a particular percentage of the sample above or below it.

Per protocol—analysis strategy in which only subjects who followed the study protocol completely are analyzed. For example, the analysis includes only subjects who got the full intervention or who got none of the intervention.

Person, place, time—components of a descriptive epidemiologic study that focus on the "who, when, and where" of the health phenomena of interest.

Plausibility—criteria for causality requiring that it must be biologically possible that an exposure can cause an outcome.

Population attributable risk—ratio of the difference between the incidence or prevalence of the total study population and that of the unexposed group to the prevalence or incidence of the total population. It is typically interpreted as the proportion or percentage of the incidence or prevalence of the outcome in the total group that can be attributed to the exposure.

Population source—broad collection, possibly national, of individuals who may be eligible as cases (e.g., cancer registries) and controls (e.g., national surveys) for case-control studies.

Poster—visual graphic presentation of study results that can be examined by an audience with or without interaction with the investigator.

Posttest—measurement of subjects after an intervention hypothesized to prevent or treat an outcome.

Power—the probability that a hypothesis test correctly rejects a false null hypothesis. The power is $(1 - \beta)$ or $(1 - p$ [Type II error]).

Power analysis—analysis used to determine the appropriate sample size for being able to detect specific meaningful results. This is the sample size that is just large enough to show meaningful results that are statistically significant.

Predictive validity—ability of a measure to predict something it should, theoretically, be able to predict.

Pretest—measurement of subjects before an intervention hypothesized to prevent or treat an outcome.

Prevalence—proportion of individuals who have a disease or some outcome during a specific point or period of time. These are existing, not new, cases at the time of the study.

Primary source—original research papers that are written by the researchers who authored the study or are responsible for designing the study. Also, data that were collected by the researcher who analyzed them.

Probability—an estimate of the likelihood that an event will occur.

Probability sampling—a sampling method with which subjects are selected using a probability-based method. The probability of selection for each subject is a known non-zero value.

Problem statement—justification of the value and purpose of the proposed research questions and hypotheses.

Program announcement (PA)—general, often ongoing, request for research proposals. Announcements are usually quite broad in focus to encourage research on a variety of related topics.

Proposal—detailed presentation of a novel study idea including the problem statement, purpose, methodology, and requested budget and personnel.

Prospective—looking forward in time. In the context of study design, a prospective cohort study first measures the exposure and then the outcome forward in time.

Protocol—document containing a detailed description of all steps and components of a particular study's procedures.

Publication bias—mistaken belief about the general relationships and phenomena in a field of study resulting from the tendency of journal editors to publish the results of studies that support hypotheses rather than those of studies that cannot support their hypotheses. Publication bias is a key issue in meta-analysis.

PubMed—searchable database of more than 21 million citations for biomedical research.

Purposive sample—procedure to identify potential subjects with predefined characteristics.

p-value—exact value of the probability of committing a Type I error or the statistical significance.

Quartiles—values on a continuous variable that separate the four quarters (25% groups) of the frequency distribution.

Quasi-experimental design—study design where subjects are not randomly assigned to treatment and control groups.

Quota sample—sample created by choosing subjects until a predetermined number of subjects with predefined characteristics have been included.

Randomization—assignment of subjects to study groups using a probability-based scheme for the purpose of minimizing systematic differences between groups.

Randomized controlled trial—experiment or evaluation design in which subjects are randomly assigned to comparison groups (i.e., experimental and control) and then followed to determine the presumed efficacy of the intervention.

Random selection—procedure for choosing subjects where all subjects have an equal probability of being selected.

Range—measure of dispersion calculated by subtracting the minimum from the maximum values of a continuous variable.

Rank—number that indicates a relative order.

Rate—the likelihood of an event occurring (e.g., dying) in a particular period of time.

Rate ratio—ratio of incidence densities (rates) for two independent groups (i.e., exposed and unexposed).

Rating scale—scaling technique for which an ordered series of category choices are listed on a numeric continuum.

Ratio level or scales—a type of continuous variable whose values are intervals with a true zero point.

Raw data—collection of data points for each subject and each measure. The data are not grouped into variables.

Recall bias—distortion in the relationship between the exposure and outcome due to one group being better able to remember an exposure compared to another (e.g., cases may be more motivated than controls to remember the exposure).

Recode—procedure to combine or change the order of variable response options.

Recognition factor—level of recognition of a particular journal in a specific field of study.

Recruitment—identifying and persuading subjects to participate in a research study.

Regression analysis—procedure to test the relationship between one or more independent or exposure variables and one dependent or outcome variables.

Regression coefficient—estimate of the parameter measuring the strength and direction of the association between one or more independent or exposure variables and an outcome or dependent variable. The coefficient is interpreted as the change in y (dependent variable) with one unit increase in x (independent variable).

Relative frequency—the number of subjects in a particular group (i.e., variable value or category) divided by the total number of subjects in the sample. The value is often expressed as a percent.

Relative risk—ratio of prevalence or incidence in the exposed group to the prevalence or incidence in the unexposed group.

Reliability (precision)—ability of a measurement instrument to give consistent results with repeated measurements.

Request for application (RFA)—specific announcements of research opportunities that may or may not reoccur. Each RFA differs in the scope of the project and the size of the potential awards. Many of these projects require multidisciplinary and multi-institutional response.

Research—investigation or experimentation aimed at the discovery and interpretation of facts.

Research question—concise, interrogative statements that guide all aspects of the study design. The questions can explore and describe phenomena, test relationships between variables, and investigate the causes of health outcomes.

Respondent—term for a research subject in a survey study.

Respondent-driven sampling—variation of snowball sampling where potential subjects are identified for the purpose of recruitment by asking subjects who meet study criteria to recruit other eligible subjects by referring them to study personnel.

Retention—act of including baseline subjects in follow-up data collections. Procedure for retaining subjects in cohort and experimental studies.

Retrospective—looking backward in time. In the context of study design, a retrospective cohort study first measures the outcome and then uses historical data to go back in time and measure the exposure.

Risk-benefit assessment—judgment made by the IRB concerning the potential risks and benefits to research subjects in a proposed study. Four relevant criteria for the assessment are: (1) risks to subjects are reasonable in relation to anticipated benefits; (2) risks to subjects are minimized; (3) when appropriate, there are adequate provisions to protect the privacy of subjects; and (4) when appropriate, the research plan makes adequate provisions for ongoing monitoring for subject safety.

Risk difference—absolute of effect of an exposure on an outcome measured by subtracting the prevalence or incidence of the unexposed group from the prevalence or incidence of the exposed group.

Risk factor—exposure that is associated with an adverse health outcome. The risk factor must precede the outcome in time.

Risk ratio—prevalence or incidence of the outcome for the exposed group divided by the prevalence or incidence of the outcome for the unexposed group. Typically interpreted as the relative difference (higher or lower) in the prevalence or incidence in the exposed compared to unexposed group.

***R*-square**—statistic calculated in regression analysis. It is the proportion of variance in the dependent variable that can be explained by the independent variable(s).

Sample—group of subjects who are a subset of the population. The goal of inferential statistics is to choose a sample that accurately represents the population.

Sample population (study population)—subset of the target population to which the researcher has access.

Sampling frame—list of individuals in the population who are available to be sampled for a study.

Sampling method—strategy for choosing subjects from a population into a sample.

Scales—unidimensional measures of multidimensional concepts. Scales are created by combining variables in some manner to represent multiple components of a concept.

Scatter plots—graphical display in which the pair of data points for each subject (i.e., the particular values for variable x and variable y) are represented by a point on a plot of the possible joint values of x and y.

Scientific method—procedure for conducting research by following the steps: (1) observe and describe health phenomena, (2) formulate a hypothesis to explain the phenomena, (3) test the hypothesis in a research study, (4) replicate the hypothesis in additional studies.

Screening—taking appropriate measures of potential subjects to determine if they meet the inclusionary criteria and do not meet the exclusionary criteria for the study.

Secondary data analysis—analysis of previously collected data (i.e., data collected by others and possibly for other purposes).

Secondary source—publications or reports that summarize or present results from primary sources.

Selection bias—distortion in the association between the exposure and outcome due to a problem in the selection of subjects for the study. The association between the exposure and outcome may be different for members of the population who participated in the study compared to those who did not participate.

Self-determination—ability of a research subject to behave in a way that she chooses.

Semantic differentials scale—response options presented on a visual continuum with two defined endpoints and simple numbers in between; usually a seven-point scale is used between the two endpoints.

Semi-structured questions—questions with a predetermined range of responses and open-ended options to elicit responses in subjects' own words.

Simple random sample—type of probability sample for which individuals are selected from the population using a random method where each individual has an equal probability of being selected.

Simple regression—technique used to estimate the equation that best describes the association between one independent or exposure variable and one dependent or outcome variable. Simple regression can be either linear (continuous outcome) or logistic (dichotomous outcome).

Skewness—measure of the degree and direction of asymmetry in a frequency distribution (i.e., the extent to which the distribution is not symmetric on either side of the mean.

Slope (*b*)—regression coefficient in a linear regression equation that measures the change in the outcome or dependent variable (*y*) with each unit change in the exposure or dependent variable (*x*).

Snowball sampling—procedure to identify potential subjects by asking subjects who meet inclusionary criteria to recommend others similar to them.

Social cognitive theory—explains how individuals acquire particular behavior patterns. Concepts of the theory include the environment, situation, behavioral capability, self-efficacy, observational learning, and more. The theory is used in public health for designing health education programs.

Social ecological model—postulates that health behaviors are influenced by the interaction between an individual and her environment. The model proposes five levels of influences—individual, interpersonal, organizational, community and social structure, and policy and systems—on health and health behavior.

Specific aims—succinct statement and description of the research goals of a proposed study.

Specificity—criteria for causality stipulating that the association between exposure and outcome is specific to particular persons, places, times, and/or health phenomena.

Standard deviation—measure of dispersion that is the square root of the sum of the squared distance of each data point from the sample mean.

Standard error—standard deviation of the sampling distribution of a statistic. It is the value that is added to and subtracted from a statistic to calculate the confidence interval around the statistic as an estimate of the population parameter.

Standard normal distribution—normal (bell-shaped) distribution with a mean of zero (0) and a standard deviation of one (1).

Statistic—summary measure computed in a sample.

Statistical power—the probability that a hypothesis test correctly rejects a false null hypothesis. The power is $(1 - \beta)$, or $(1 - p$ [Type II error]).

Statistical significance—represented by the *p*-value in the hypothesis test. A result is said to be statistically significant if the *p*-value is less than or equal to the predetermined alpha (α) value meaning that the result is unlikely to be due to chance.

Stratification—procedure for separating subjects into mutually exclusive or nonoverlapping groups or strata.

Stratified random sample—a type of probability sample for which subjects are selected randomly from mutually exclusive or nonoverlapping groups or strata of the population.

STROBE—acronym for Strengthening the Reports of Observational Studies in Epidemiology, which provides guidelines for reporting the results of observational studies (cohort, case-control, and cross-sectional).

Structured questions—questions with a predetermined range of responses for the respondent to select.

Study-by-study review—type of literature review that summarizes the main components of each study, one at a time, according to a specific theme of the review.

Sum of squares—statistic calculated in ANOVA. It is the sum of squared deviations for the model (each group mean from the total mean), error (each data point from its respective group mean), or total (sum of the model and error sums).

Survey—type of data collection method that involves asking questions.

Survival analysis—methods used to analyze outcomes measured as the amount of time until an event (e.g., disease or death) occurs.

Symmetry—situation in which the shape of a frequency distribution is the same on either side of the mean. For example, a normal distribution is symmetric on either side of the mean.

Systematic random sample—a type of probability sample for which subjects are chosen from a sampling frame at a predetermined interval in the list of individuals defined by $k = N/n$, where N is the size of the population (or sampling frame) and n is the desired size of the sample being selected.

Systematic review—in-depth literature review with the purpose of identifying, reviewing, and synthesizing all empirical evidence that meets the prespecified eligibility criteria.

Target or theoretical population—entire group to which a study strives to generalize results.

Temporality—timing of the occurrence of the exposure and the outcome.

Test-retest reliability—consistency of a measure tested by conducting the measurement at two different time points and correlating the resulting measures.

Test statistic—summary measure used to determine the statistical significance in hypothesis tests. Example are Z, t, χ^2, and F.

Thematic review—type of literature review that focuses on a theme and, in a succinct manner, cites multiple studies to document important findings under each theme. The focus is mainly on discussing the main findings or results of the studies that address the theme rather than reviewing several components of each study.

Theory—set of principles or statements to explain a phenomenon that has been addressed with multiple hypotheses and research questions.

Timeline—schedule for completing all phases of the study in the requested time period of funding. The timeline names and defines each step in the research process and estimates how long each will take to complete.

Transtheoretical model—model of behavior change based on the conception of stages of change (pre-contemplation, contemplation, preparation, action, and maintenance), which influence the degree of readiness to adopt healthful behaviors.

t **score**—test statistic for hypothesis tests using continuous measures with a relatively small ($n < 30$) sample size.

Tuskegee Syphilis Study—40-year study of the natural history of syphilis among 600 mostly poor and uneducated black men in Tuskegee, Alabama. Even with the general acceptance of penicillin as an effective treatment of syphilis in 1947, the men were not offered this treatment.

Type I error—rejecting a null hypothesis that is really true.

Type II error—failing to reject a null hypothesis that is really false.

Unit of observation—single entity from which data are collected.

Univariate—analysis of a single variable using descriptive statistics.

Validity (accuracy)—ability of a measure to give a true result and to measure the concept it is intended to measure.

Variable—analyzable measure that has two or more categories across which subjects are distributed.

Variance—measure of dispersion that is the sum of the squared distance of each data point from the sample mean.

Voluntary consent—decision to participate in a research study made without coercion or undue influence.

Willowbrook Hepatitis Study—research conducted in 1956 where mentally disabled children at the Willowbrook State School in New York were injected with the hepatitis A virus to study the immunity response in pursuit of an effective vaccine.

Z **score**—test statistic for hypothesis tests using continuous measures with a relatively large ($n \geq 30$) sample size.

INDEX

A

abstract, 237–238, 246, 251–252
active follow-up data collection, 147
African American women, hypothetical
    breast cancer study, 116
alpha, 126
ambispective cohort designs, 42–43
American Journal of Public Health, 241
analysis of variance (ANOVA), 184, 188,
    196, 210, 228
associative research study, 10–17
    confounding in, 12–14
    effect modification (interaction), 14–15
    Framingham Heart Study, 15–17
    measures of association test relationships
        between exposures and outcomes,
        11–12
    risk factors, identifying, 11
attributable risk (AR), 12
attrition bias, 126, 146

B

Behavior Risk Factor Surveillance System
    (BRFSS), 153
Belmont Report, 58
beneficence, 54–58
benefits from research, 63–64
beta, 126–127

bias, 46, 63, 141, 216
    attrition, 126, 146
    classification, 45
    minimizing/preventing, steps for, 45–46
    misclassification, 40
    nonresponse, 124–125
    in the process of obtaining subjects, 125
    publication, 98–99, 199
    selection, 40, 124
birth data, 152
blinding, 46–47
Box-Whisker Plot, 177–178
breast cancer study, sampling for, 115–116
budget and budget justification for research
    study, 248–249

C

call-outs, 228
cardiovascular disease (CVD) risk
    factors, 76
case-control studies, 40–41, 47
    clinical source for cases, 40–41
    of colorectal cancer, 76
    features of design, 40
    HIV cases, examples, 41–42
    of HIV cases in Belgium, case
        example, 41–42
    selection of cases, 40